The Vagus

TABLE OF CONTENTS

INTRODUCTION

The human body is a system as intricate as there ever was. Out of all the complexities of the modern world, the ingenuity of our inventions and the wonders of the universe, the human body is still a masterpiece. From the moments we started we learn to nurse ourselves, which I don't believe anybody can provide a time for, to the early days of modern medicine, which I believe started when we started to intelligently consider internal organs and their roles in the body, to medicine today, our body can still surprise us.

In all the surprises that the body will throw at us, we are certain of one thing, every organ in the human body are there for a reason even the ones we can lose have their functions.

The idea of every organ of the body needing each other and working together is not strange. We have known that before science.

What we didn't know know is how they communicate. Science has answered that question too, the central nervous system.

The vagus nerve is a part of the central nervous system. That is not news. The Vagus nerve is a network that transmits signals between the organs of the body and the brain. Most people would wonder why they need that information.

When I say that the vagus nerve can be used to explain many psychological and physiological health conditions, that will get some people's attention. Then when I or any other person, professional health care provider or an average Joe say that the vagus nerve can be to heal the body, that will grab attention but only a few number if people will actually listen.

I also didn't sit up and listen the first time I heard it, but today here I am writing a book about the vagus nerve.

This book is brief and nontechnical. I wrote it with the newbie in mind. It is intended to introduce you to the vagus nerve and teach you how to harness the power of an organ that is so mysterious yet connected to various organs of the body and involved with many bodily functions.

This book is about a safe , cheap and efficient healing practice. It is about using the vagus nerve's network and connection to influence and heal the body.

SECTION ONE

WHAT IS THE VAGUS NERVE?

Vagus is a derivative of the Latin word or "rambling, wandering or uncertain." The name was chosen due to the enigma of the vagus nerve. Anatomists can tell exactly what it is, but they know that the nerve wanders to many parts of the body.

The vagus nerve starts from the brainstem, the regulator of the autonomic nervous system. The brainstem senses, processes and regulates most of body's automatic functions. Automatic functions are the ones that our body performs automatically and unconsciously. Examples of automatic functions include:

- Sexual arousal
- Sweating
- Digestion
- Breathing

- Production of tears and saliva

- Detoxification of the kidney and liver

- Dilation of blood vessels

- Dilation of the pupils

The brainstems contain numerous groups of neurons called nuclei (nucleus for singular). The neurons are responsible for transmitting information to various parts of the body. They take information to and from the brain. There are two major types of neurons based on the direction information is being transmitted to. They are called afferent neurons and efferent neurons. Afferent neurons transmit information from the body to the brain while efferent neurons transmit information from the brain to other parts of the body. Efferent information, is information transmitted by efferent neurons are called consist motor and regulatory information.

Most of the nerves in the body carry simple motor signals or sensory information around the body. The vagus nerve performs much more than that. The left and right part of the vagus nerve contains four separate nuclei, each one with a different function. Of all the information carried by the neurons of the vagus nerve, about 20% are efferent information while the remaining 80% are afferent information. This means that most of the information in the vagus nerve is moving from the body to the brain. The vagus nerve transmits four times more information to the brain than it transmits away from it. Even with this, the efferent information it transmits is enough to have a huge impact on different organs.

Neurons are like a wired network, the information is transmitted like an electric signal which releases a chemical signal called neurotransmitter at the end of the line. The neurotransmitter then triggers an effect on the receiving cell by binding with a receptor on the receiving cell.

The vagus nerve mainly uses Acetylcholine (Ach), a neurotransmitter with an anti-inflammatory effect. This makes regulating inflammation a major function of the vagus nerve. In fact, the vagus nerve is the body's main manager of inflammation. Inflammation is the body's response to infections. It is a self-defense mechanism that sometimes gets out of hand. When inflammation becomes acute, it can lead to several health conditions. Some of the health conditions that may be caused by inflammation include:

- Diabetes
- High blood pressure
- Cancer
- Alzheimer's disease
- Heart disease
- Arthritis
- High cholesterol levels

All the organs affected in these conditions are connected to the Vagus nerve. It would be simplistic and dangerous to attribute these health conditions to the Vagus nerve and inflammation alone. There are many other factors that may contribute to these diseases but the contributions of inflammation cannot be ignored.

The anatomy of the vagus nerve

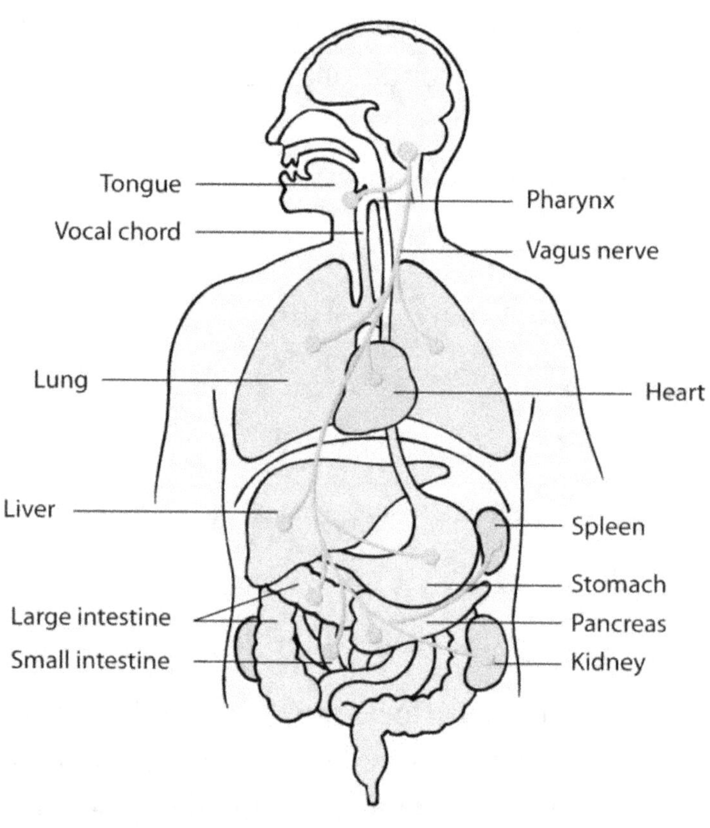

The Brainstem- the starting point

The vagus nerve consists of neurons that begin at the brainstems. These neurons make up four nuclei. Each one of the nuclei control different fibers of the vagus nerve. The four nuclei are:

- Spinal trigeminal nucleus

Signals from the exterior part of the body transmitted through the skin by sensory neurons are transported through the vagus nerve by the spinal trigeminal nucleus.

- Nucleus solitarius (solitary nucleus)

Internal signals are transported by the vagus nerve to the nucleus solitarius (solitary nucleus). Internal signals are signals from internal organs such as the liver, intestine, heart, lungs, spleen, gallbladder, stomach and pancreas.

- Dorsal motor nucleus

The vagus nerve also sends signals to these organs through the dorsal motor nucleus. These signals control and regulate the aforementioned organs.

- Nucleus ambiguus.

The vagus nerve sends out neurons that possesses a motor function through the nucleus ambiguous. These neurons control most of the muscles in our upper airway and throat. They keep the airway open and vocal, ensuring our ability to speak/make sounds with our mouth.

The Neck

The fibers of the right and left sections of the vagus nerve extend from the medulla oblongata to the cranial cavity, where they converge into the vagus nerve. The vagus nerve exits the skull through the jugular foramen, a large opening between the skull and the neck that nerves and blood vessels pass through.

The vagus nerve leaves the skull for an area in the upper neck, behind the ear and between the internal carotid artery and internal jugular vein. Jugular/superior ganglion occurs as soon as the vagus nerve passes through the jugular foramen. It is the thickening of the vagus nerve by the sensory neuron cells. The cell bodies join to form a thinner nerve section, resulting in the first branch of the vagus nerve.

This branch is called the auricular branch. It returns to the skull through the mastoid canaliculus and comes back out of the skull and heads for the ear through the tympanomastoid fissure. It then extends through the skin of the ears. The auricular branch or the vagus nerve senses temperature, touch and moisture/wetness on the skin of the air, especially the auricle, tragus and external canal.

The vagus nerve thickens again to form the inferior/nodose ganglion, as it moves downward. The neurons in the inferior ganglion transmit information from internal organs.

The vagus nerve thins back and passes through a passageway made by the thickening of the carotid sheath (a connecting tissue).

The vagus nerve forms another branch in the in the carotid sheath. This new branch is called the pharyngeal branch. It contains neurons from the vagus nerve, the glossopharyngeal nerves (ninth cranial nerves) and the accessory nerves (eleventh cranial nerves).

The pharyngeal branch moves through the midline of the body until the reach the pharynx (the upper throat). Here, they release motor signals to the muscles responsible for opening and closing the mouth, gag reflex and swallowing.

The vagus nerve forms another branch called the superior laryngeal nerve as it moves down the carotid sheath on the sides of the neck. The superior laryngeal nerve transmits motor signals to the muscles that control the pitch of the voice and other muscles of the larynx, above the vocal chords.

The vagus nerve forms another branch called the thoracic cardiac branch. It is formed after passing through the carotid sheath in the chest. It supplies sensory signals to the heart. It mingles with some nerves of the nervous system to form cardiac plexus.

The Thorax

The vagus nerve continues downward into the thorax after leaving the carotid sheath. The left vagus nerve travels in front of the arch of the aorta and another laryngeal branch is formed. The right vagus nerve travels in front of the right subclavian artery and also forms a laryngeal nerve. Both laryngeal branches go upward, towards the neck. They transmit motor signals to the larynx muscles below the vocal cords. This helps to loosen and tension the vocal chords in order to produce sound.

Both the left and right vagus nerves send another branch to the lungs. The right vagus nerve sends a pulmonary branch to the posterior pulmonary plexus while the left vagus nerve sends a pulmonary branch to the anterior pulmonary plexus. They mingle with some neurons and connect to the bronchi on each lung.

The vagus nerve also transmits signals to and fro the thymus. The thymus is a vital part of the immune system that is located between the sternum and the heart. It is responsible for the training and growth of white blood cells. It develops early but may be covered by fat tissue as we age.

The Abdomen

The vagus nerve also innervates the abdomen, which aids digestion, detoxification and the entire immune system. The first branch extends to the stomach where it stimulates the stomach muscles for digestion. They also stimulate the stomach's muscle cells to push and churn the food and the parietal cells to produce hydrochloric acid (HCI), which is responsible for the secretion of digestive enzymes like gastrin and renin.

The second branch extends to the liver, where it may help generate hunger and craving for some nutrients. We absorb most macronutrients such as amino acid, carbohydrates, fat into the bloodstream in the small intestine. The nutrients then pass through the portal vein into the liver where they are filtered, detoxified and processed while the vagus nerve transmits signals to the brain. This signal involves details of fat intake, liver functionality, blood sugar level and quantity of bile needed in the digestion of fat.

The gallbladder holds the bile and bile salt created by liver in readiness of another meal. The vagus nerve helps the gallbladder pump the bile into the duodenum when we are eating. This process releases fat into the bloodstream. It is activated when the taste buds sense fat in the food.

Another branch is extended to the pancreas and transmits message to and fro the brain. The pancreas has endocrine and exocrine parts. The exocrine pancreas secretes digestive enzymes into the small intestine. The most popular of these enzymes are amylase (for breaking down carbohydrates), lipase (for breaking down fat), and protease (for breaking down protein). The endocrine pancreas balances the glucose levels by secreting glucagon and insulin into the bloodstream.

The vagus nerve transmits information about endocrine and exocrine cells from the pancreas to the brain. It also transmits information from the brain to the pancreas, about food content and the enzymes to be released into the digestive system and the bloodstream.

After the stomach, the parasympathetic fibers of the vagus combine with the lumbar sympathetic nerves to form the celiac plexus, a network that extends branches to the remaining organs of the abdomen.

It first branches into the spleen on the left side of the body, where it monitors the bloodstream and controls the immune system. The spleen shares the responsibility of controlling the immune system with the thymus until the thymus starts to disappear as we grow up.

Then it extends to the small intestine where it triggers the transportation of food down the tract. The digested food is passed into the small intestine where it undergoes further digestion. The vagus nerve triggers the smooth muscle cells of the gut to push a chyme (technical name for a bite of food) down the digestive tract.

The vagus also extends to the large intestine, where it transmits signals between the brain and the large intestine. The large intestine hosts the symbiotic bacterial that live in our gut. These bacterial produce biochemical precursors, minerals and vitamins. They also produce harmful gasses and toxins. The vagus nerve helps the body to keep the microbiome in check by transmitting information about the microbiome to the brain and instructions back to the large intestine.

Lastly, the vagus nerve extends into the kidneys. It helps the kidney to maintain pressure which is needed to filter fluid out of the body. The fluid is urine, a combination of water and uric acid.

The vagus nerve ends by combining with the parasympathetic nerves at the lower end of the spine. This network innervates the descending and sigmoid colon (the second half of the large intestine), the sex organs and the bladder.

WHAT DOES THE VAGUS NERVE DO?

The vagus nerve is essential in the maintenance of a healthy and fully functional human body. It is like a communication network that spreads that connects different organs to the control center (the brain), hereby ensuring smooth well-oiled operation. The wrong signals and misinformation between organs can have disastrous consequences. It is also more than a message network because it triggers actions in different organs. It regulates the functions of organs and ensures uniformity of their action. Here are the major functions that the vagus nerve performs in the body.

It allows us to feel sensation in the skin of the ear

The vagus nerve allows us to feel touch, wetness and temperature on the skin of the tragus, auricle and the external auditory canal of the ear. These parts are located in the central sections of the ear and acupuncture is taking advantage by using these locations to stimulate the vagus nerve.

It manages the vocal chords and airway

The vagus nerve is responsible for opening the upper airway and making it possible to breathe and speak or make any noise with our mouth. The superior laryngeal (the third branch of the vagus nerve) controls the muscle above the vocal chords by transmitting motor signals to the muscles. This controls the vocal chords and changes the pitch of our voices. The irritation of the vagus nerve can result in hoarse or feeble voice and in extreme cases increase the possibility of asphyxiation and severe cough.

The recurrent laryngeal (the fourth branch of the vagus nerve) controls the muscles below the chord. The motor signal it carries to these muscles allow the vocal chords to tension, open and close. It also has a sensory ability that allows it to relay transmit signal to the trachea and esophagus.

If the recurrent laryngeal is irritated, it can make a person lose their voice or cause the voice to become hoarse. It can also cause breathing problems.

It manages the liver and its functions

The liver alone performs hundreds of functions in the body, with around 500 duties, it is no lightweigh. One of these functions, the one I am currently interested in is the regulating of the blood flow throughout the body. The arms are legs are prioritized when the body enters fight or flight mode, therefore blood is diverted to them. This activates the muscles and gives the arms and legs the strength required to take the appropriate action. It also cause a decrease in the flow of blood in the liver but it doesn't matter because the filtration and digestion are not prioritized at that moment. The process is reversed when the body returns to rest mode. Filtration and digestion becomes a priority again and the blood flow to the liver is increased.

The liver also produces bile and bile salt which are transported to the gallbladder and small intestine. The vagus nerve indirectly controls both the production and the transportation of bile and bile salt. Experts have noticed that cholangiocytes, the cells responsible for both actions are active when the vagus nerve is active. The vagus nerve activates the cholangiocytes cells and to produce the bile and bile salt then transport it to the small intestine.

The liver's detoxification of fat-soluble toxins to create water-soluble waste is undertaken in two stages. One of the duties of the bile is to hold the stool, which contains some of the waste products. The rest of these waste products are held in our sweats and urine.

Bile salts on the other hand, move with fat molecules from the digestive system and through the enterocytes cells (lining the small intestine) into the bloodstream. Fat can only be absorbed in the presence of bile salt and they will likely end up in the stool, causing fatty stool. The fat is also important to the body.

It manages our breathing

The vagus nerve innervates the trachea and bronchi of the lungs through the pulmonary branch which connect to the pulmonary plexus of the nervous system. It transmits information from the lungs to the brain about the oxygen, CO2 and lung expansion levels. The vagus nerve can make the breath shallow or deep.

When a person is in the rest mode, the breathing is usually deep and slow, the breath rises from the diaphragm. The breath is shallow and fast when in a fight or flight mode but it begins to slow down as the person transitions to rest mode.

The vagus nerve is responsible for the opening and closing of the trachea, larynx and pharynx. This is accomplished through the transmission of motor actions. If the vagus nerve is not performing these functions properly, it can obstruct the airway. These may ultimately lead to obstructive sleep apnea and Chronic Obstructive Pulmonary Disease (COPD).

It maintains our blood pressure

The vagus nerve transmit information to and fro the kidneys to aid the control of fluids and water flowing into the bloodstream. The kidney filters the fluids and water using the kidney glomeruli, and removes toxins from the body, herby maintaining the blood pressure. The blood vessels send signals to the brain when the body is under stress. The brainstem then transmits signals to the kidney, through the vagus nerves. The signals trigger the kidney to increase the blood pressure. The kidney accomplishes this by constricting its blood vessels to reduce the quantity of water it filters out of the bloodstream.

This process is reversed when the body is starts returning to rest mode. The kidney receives signals to increase the quantity of water it filters out of the blood stream. The vagus nerve and sympathetic nerves are not solely responsible for these actions, as the hormones are also involved.

A dysfunctional vagus nerve can cause over-activation of the stress hormones in the adrenal glands which couples with the immune autonomic system's response to it to result in high blood pressure and hypertension.

It controls our heart rate

The vagus nerve ensures that the heartbeat is at a comfortable rate. The activities of the vagus nerve help the heart generate the right reaction to situations and avoid stress. The beating of the heart allows it to pump blood into body cells and move toxins to organs that will store and dispose them. The vagus nerve connects to the sinoatrial node, a tissue that sends electrical signals to the two thinner chambers of the heart (the atria), and the atrioventricular node, a tissue that controls the pumping rate and contraction pressure of the two larger chambers of the heart (the ventricles). Each connection is separate and direct.

The vagus nerve stimulates the nervous system to make the heart increase the pressure of the contraction of the ventricles, thus increasing the heart rate, when in fight or flight mode. The situation is reverse when the body is returning to rest mode, the heart is activated to reduce the pressure of the contraction of the ventricles and decrease the heart rate.

It activates the Gallbladder to empty its contents

The gallbladder is like a save that holds bile until it is required during digestion of the next meal. The taste buds transmit signals to the brain, when you eat. These signals also contain information about the macronutrients they sensed in every bite of the food. If fat is being consumed, the central nervous system transmits signals to the liver and the gallbladder which prepares to release fat into the small intestine.

The gallbladder then activates the smooth muscle walls that line it, after receiving the alert signal. The muscle walls will pump bile into the small intestine through the bile duct. This signal is transmitted by the vagus nerve and without it the gallbladder wouldn't know when to empty the gall bladder. The gallbladder then becomes and remains full resulting in a medical condition called the obstructive cholestasis. Obstructions due to gallstone are one of the most common medical conditions that affect the gallbladder. The resulting surgery to remove the gallstones is one of the most common surgeries performed annually in the United States. The surgery is called cholecystectomy and it is usually recommended when patients begin to feel pain resulting from obstructions like gallstones. Gallstones are painful and it takes a while for them to form in the gallbladder. This is usually due to long term dysfunction of the vagus nerve. A dysfunctional vagus nerve results in the gallbladder not transporting the bile and bile duct out. They tend start to crystalline and form stones, the longer they remain in the gallbladder.

This condition is one of the earliest effects of a dysfunctional vagus nerve, it also doesn't exactly require surgery to fix although surgery has been the common route. The gallbladder can remove the gallstones, if it starts functioning optimally. Some exercise that will help you activate the gallbladder will be provided in this book. It is the aim of this book, we are not just here to talk about the vagus nerve. I intend to show you how to activate it.

It controls satiety and hunger

When we are satisfied with food and hunger is quenched, the vagus nerve transmits this signal the brain. The liver is the main organ in this task. It transmits signals through the vagus nerve to the brain, that we have consumed enough protein, carbohydrate and fat. The liver metabolizes carbohydrate and fat.

The vagus nerve indirectly transmits signals to the brain, indicating that we need more carbohydrates when the blood sugar level is low. When the body is satiated, the small intestine releases peptide 1 (GLP-1), which is very similar to glucagon. This is how the body is notified to satiety. The presence of peptide 1 is increased in the bloodstream. When the amount of peptide 1 in the bloodstream is reduced, it also reduces the blood sugar levels. After each meal the vagus nerve transmits information to the brain about the quantity of triglycerides, linoleic acid and other fats that made it into the liver. The vagus nerve then curbs hunger by transmitting a signal which generates satiety to the brain. With a fully functionally vagus nerve

A dysfunction vagus nerve won't perform this duty adequately. This may result in constant hunger and overeating.

It aids in the swallowing of food

The pharyngeal branch of the vagus nerve, allow us to swallow food unconsciously. It controls two muscles that connect the soft palate to the throat and three constrictor muscles at the back of the throat. These muscles push the chyme to the larynx and esophagus. This allows us to swallow food. It also keeps the food away from the trachea (keeping the airway clear) and pause the breathing reflex after each bite to prevent us from choking.

The pharyngeal branch also manages the gag reflex, meaning that we can manipulate the vagus nerve using the gag reflex.

It controls the motor function of the digestive tract

The digestive tract is a long and intricate pathway consisting of various organs. Food must move from one end of the digestive tract (the mouth) until the waste material (stool, urine and sweat) are removed from the body.

All these movements are stimulated by the vagus nerve. When we take a bite of food, we usually chew it until it can be swallowed. After swallowing the food is transported through the lengths of the digestive tract. The first step is the pharynx, which is located at the back of the throat. The autonomous system take control, as every action from this point is subconscious. The vagus nerve takes control. It triggers the smooth muscles lining the walls of the gut to push the food. Every bite generates a reaction from the muscles which in turn transmits a signal to the brain. The brain replies back with a signal to start motor actions and push the food down the gut. The process is called peristalsis and the vagus nerve is the medium when information is transmitted in both directions. The long journey through the gut allows the body to extract nutrients from the food and separate unwanted constituents. This activity and the length of the gut make the process more complex than it looks.

A dysfunctional vagus nerve results in a disruption of this process. The muscles and nerves are impaired, and it can result in diarrhea and chronic constipation. A simple and common cause of this dysfunction is not chewing the food properly and rushing your food. The rest mode is essential for digestion but most people in the modern world eat their food in the fight of flight mode. The body prioritizes action over digestion in this stance and the digestive process suffers.

It controls the release of digestive enzymes from the Pancreas

The pancreas produces and secretes digestive enzymes into the small intestine. The sensory intestinal cells and taste buds of the tongue transmit a signal to the brain. This signal contains information about the macronutrients present in the food. This include how much and how fast fat, carbohydrate and protein where consumed. The information is used to determine the kind of digestive enzyme required and the quantity in which they are needed. These enzymes (for example amylase, lipase and protease) are required to digest the ingested food and they also help to optimize the usage of the basic nutrients generated from the digested food.

If the food contains fat, the pancreas secretes lipase which breaks down the fat into triglycerides and free fatty acid. If the food contains protein, it secretes protease which breaks the protein into amino acids. If the food contains carbohydrate, the pancreas secrets amylase which breakdowns the carbohydrates to simple sugars.

The simple forms can then be absorbed by the body and use to facilitate cell functions. Amino acids are used by the cells to produce protein, receptors, peptide hormones, intracellular signaling molecules and neurotransmitters. Simple sugar and free fatty acids are the main resources for producing energy. Cholesterol is functions as a precursor for steroid hormones like, cortisol, testosterone and estrogen. Every one of these is required for optimal functionality of the human body. A dysfunction in any department can set of a cycle of disaster.

It manages the insulin and blood sugar levels

Some of the most rampant health problems today include obesity and diabetes. This two problems are a result of an unhealthy lifestyle resulting in weight problems and blood sugar level problems, respectively.

When the human body is under stress, the body activates fight or flight mode. This mode is a result of evolution and a deeply ingrained instead developed from the earlier days of man, when most of the creatures on earth were larger than him. Flight was the major option until fight also became more prominent. These two, fight or flight are our response to a threat. When the body is in fight of flight mode, the balance shifts to the sympathetic nervous system and more adrenaline is released, especially cortisol. Cortisol raises the blood sugar level by instigating the creation of glucose from protein and fat available in the liver. The process is called gluconeogenesis.

The nervous system tries to funnel out energy to the essential organs and body parts required to make the next decision and act on it. The legs and ands are the main targets. These creates short term fuel, glucose in a process called gluconeogenesis and releases it into the bloodstream. Blood flow to the legs and arms are increased because they have been prioritized. The muscles of these body parts are strengthened by the increased blood flow, making the fight or flight action easier, faster and more effective.

This system may fall short in its timing by remaining active for longer than required. Due to the stressful environment of the modern world, the body is almost always in a fight or flight mode. Several modern activities from work, transportation, managing our finances and even some mundane daily activities contribute to the stressful environment. This situation leaves the body in constant stress and reduces the amount of time spent in rest and digest mode. The liver keeps producing glucose hereby increasing the blood sugar levels at an unhealthy rate and on a long term.

The body reacts to this by trying to reduce the amount of glucose in the blood. This is accomplished by triggering the pancreas to produce insulin, a chemical that signals the cells of the body to absorb glucose from the blood and convert it to energy. As this is a long term problem the pancreas keep producing insulin and the insulin keeps signaling the cells of the body to absorb glucose from the blood. Over time the cells become resistant to insulin and they begin to reject the messages. After other cells have stopped absorbing glucose from the blood, the adipocytes (adipose tissue) is the only one that keeps absorbing the glucose and it receives all the messages from the insulin and absorbs as many glucose as it can. The adipose tissue is also called the fat tissue and it can be found in every part of the body although it is mostly concentrated in the stomach. This is how people gain weight and it ultimately becomes type II diabetes. At this stage the pancreas has produced so much insulin that it became worn out. People with diabetics are usually prescribed insulin or medications that stimulate insulin sensitivity in the cells. Ultimately, high blood sugar levels can lead to obesity, insulin resistance and diabetes. The high blood sugar levels may be caused by a high sugar diet, chronic overeating and chronic stress.

The constant flight or fight mode adds to the blood sugar levels and the vagus nerve is responsible for transmitting the signal that triggers the body to return to the rest mode. Digestion is prioritized in the rest mode, so is the decrement of glucose production (gluconeogenesis) and increment of insulin sensitivity. The vagus nerve signals the liver to produce hepatic insulin sensitizing substance, a molecule that increases glucose storage in muscle cells and insulin sensitivity.

Regular activation of the vagus nerve allows the body to return to rest mode more often and decrease the production of glucose and the risk of insulin resistance.

It manages inflammation in the digestive tract

The vagus nerve transmits information about the responses of the immune system between various organs of the body and the brain. The pathway through which these signals travel is called the cholinergic anti-inflammatory pathway. The cholinergic anti-inflammatory pathway connects the cells of the autoimmune system and one of its most active locations is in the gut. It uses the neurotransmitter Acetylcholine (ACh) to transmit signals that calm the immune system in other to reduce inflammation.

The signals transmitted by the vagus nerves from the spleen and thymus to the brain increase noticeable due to the increasing production of stress chemicals such as lipopolysaccharides (LPS).LPS is a toxin generated and released into the gut by certain bacterial, pathogen and viruses. It is a good thing that the autoimmune system is constantly on alert due to the stress-inducing environment and ready to engage the invaders. The white blood cells send out a signal that is transmitted to the GALT (Gut-Associated Lymphoid tissues). This triggers the sympathetic nerves and a stress response. Adrenaline also called norepinephrine (NE), a neurotransmitter receives a signal from the sympathetic nerves. The white blood cells are then triggered by the adrenaline and they proceed to combat the invading pathogens and stressor chemicals.

This system is a very important and efficient one that requires a well-defined start and stop button or instructions. The vagus nerve performs this function it keeps the autoimmune system and the generated inflammation in check. The vagus nerve accomplishes this by transmitting ACh from the gut to the parts of the body where inflammation is building up. The ACh's job is to counteract the inflammation which is a reaction to adrenalin and the sympathetic nerves.

This makes the system, in simple terms a balance between sympathetic and parasympathetic nerves. Sympathetic nerves trigger a cycle that results in inflammation and parasympathetic nerves try to shut down inflammation after it has done its job.

The enteric nervous system also known by the alias "the second brain" elevates and improves the secretion of ACh from the gut. The enteric nervous system is a collection of nerve cells that control interactions between the central nervous system and the microbiome. It is located in the gut.

The alpha-7 nicotinic acetylcholine receptor slows down the response of the immune system and decrease the activation of ACh on white blood cells, when it is required. The alpha-7 nicotinic acetylcholine receptor is found on the surface of white blood cells.

It controls the autoimmune system

The immune system is the body's self-defense network. It protects us save from infections. It also needs to be managed and the vagus nerve does a good job of doing these. This mostly consists of transmitting the activating signal at the right time and the deactivation signal at the right time. If the immune system is not activated at the right time the infection will keep damaging the body cells, the immune system combats this. The immune system will start attacking healthy cells if it is not instructed to stop after eliminating the infection. The immune system consists of leukocytes (white blood cells), which transmit sensors that inspect the body for the likelihood of toxins and infectious pathogens. The white blood cells wander the bloodstream and denote the nutrients and other materials that enter the bloodstream. They then signal white blood cells to perform their functions and eliminate unwanted constituents and invaders.

White blood cells that discover invaders and infections near their location will assess the threat and relay SOS messages, asking for support by releasing cytokines (a form of protein), in the area. This attracts nearby white blood cells that will provide back up in combating the invading pathogens. The vagus nerve detects the cytokines (SOS messages) and relays the signal to the brain to the brain informing it about the beginning of a potential inflammation. According to recent research, the vagus nerve can differentiate between the different types of cytokines and therefore it can tell the brain the specific type of inflammation that is building up.

The immune system contains several types of white blood cells. Examples include the mast cells, the macrophages, natural killer cells, neutrophils, monocytes and dendritic cells (phagocytes such as lymphocytes, eosinophils and basophil).

The phagocytes scout toxins, dangerous proteins, harmful bacterial and dead or dying human cells. When the find these items, they begin to eat the items. That is where the name "phagocytes" comes from, it literally translate to "cells that eat." The process is known as phagocytosis. The invading constituents are broken down and the remnants are filtered out of the bloodstream into the liver and other immune organs. The different phagocytes monitor and sense different invading constituents. Their reaction to the invaders is also different.

The mast cells contain granules rich in histamine and they release them into the bloodstream. This puts them in charge of allergies such as anaphylaxis. They level of their activeness depends on the rate or number of allergies a person is dealing with. This means that the more allergic the person is, the more active the mast cells are. They are located in the brain and guts and they act by activating the symptoms of a condition. The mast cells can lead to inflammation in the brain by being hyper active and causing the brain cells and nerves to become hyper sensitive to pain. They can also cause a similar reaction in the digestive tract. Inflammation of the digestive tract can impair the movement of food.

Inflammation during a reaction by the immune system is activated by the basophils. They contribute to allergic conditions such as asthma, hay fever, anaphylaxis and atopic dermatitis. These conditions and the inflammation can be triggered by allergies, pathogens and parasites. These triggers may enter into the internal parts of the body from broken skin or the digestive tract.

Eosinophils duties are combating infections and parasites. Attacks from infections, pathogens and other parasites trigger the eosinophils to activate allergic symptoms. An overstimulation of the eosinophils can be problematic because it triggers these symptoms excessively. Eosinophils also contribute to the fight against allergies such as asthma.

Natural killer

The natural killer cells are the main white blood cells responsible for fighting growth of tumors and virus attacks. These cells have don't need a sensor to differentiate between a healthy human cell and an invading cell. When they malfunction, the natural killer cell can ironically lead to an increase growth of tumor and cancerous cells. It also impairs the body's ability to distinguish between the healthy cells and invading cell and the body's ability to attack the cancerous cells.

Antibodies (also called immunoglobulin) are the sensors that roam the bloodstream and internal organs looking for infections. They are produced by the white blood cells. The five types of antibodies and each performs a different function and work at different speed. include Immunoglobulin D (IgD), Immunoglobulin G (IgG), Immunoglobulin M (IgM), Immunoglobulin A (IgA), Immunoglobulin E (IgE). The IgE, IgM and IgD are the least common type of antibodies, they are present on the surface of the mature white blood cells and they perform functions similar to the more common IgG, which we will talk about next.

The most common antibody is the IgG, its job is to identify foreign cells and proteins and trigger a journey of autoimmune response and inflammation. The IgG can be found on the surface of mature immune cell.

The IGA is next to the IgG in terms of popularity. IgA is also called secretory IgA. It is secreted in bodily fluids such as saliva, breast milk and gut secreted fluids. It is used to sense the presence of potential threats of viruses, yeasts, bacteria and parasite in the digestive system. When there is a high presence of IgA, it indicates the presence of threats but when the presence of IgA is low, this indicates a malfunctioning immune system.

The vagus nerve maintains the immune system and keeps its actions in check. It sets off the cholinergic anti-inflammatory pathway when the presence of infections is detected. The pathway controls the immune system using the vagus nerve's connection to immune organs such as the gut, spleen and thymus.

The gut/digestive tract is the most common entry point for invading infections and pathogens. That is why the gut has the most white blood cells of any organ in the body lining the cells of the intestine. These cells are attached to the walls of the entire digestive tract. They are located in small openings in the muscle walls. These muscle tissues are called Gut-Associated Lymphoid tissues (GALT). The vagus nerve regulates the action of the white blood cells of the gut and manages the inflammatory reactions. It also transmits signals between the brain and the guts.

The spleen is like a qualifier of filter of red and white blood cells. It ensures that only matures, qualified and fully trained white blood cells enter the bloodstream and cells of the body parts and organs. It disqualifies and removes white blood cells that are not up to standard, both those that are immature and those that have started reaching the peak of optimum functions and declining in functionality. It is virtually a check and balance instigator for the body. A properly functional spleen allows the immune system to attack infections and protect the body without attacking the cells of the body. The vagus nerve transmits signals throughout the central nervous system, alerting the system to the cells that are being removed from the bloodstream and tissues. When the vagus nerve malfunctions due to the activation of sympathetic branches of the vagus nerve or chronic stress, it affects the spleen. It decreases the functionality of the spleen and hereby reduces the filtration of red and white blood cells. This allows the presence of unqualified and ineffective red and white blood cells functioning within the body. These cells cannot perform the duties required of them properly and it reduces the efficiency of the auto-immune system. It is like sending unqualified and ill-trained cops to patrol and enforce law and order in the prairie.

The thymus is a lymphatic organ that produces white blood cells (called T cells) which search for and destroy invading pathogens. The thymus develops early in man and it remains functional until it starts to reduce in size and lose its functionality when we attain puberty. Experts have recently discovered that the constant fight or flight mod and stressful environment of the modern world can reduce the time span of the thymus and cause it to rescind early. The rescindment of the thymus in size and functionality is called the "involution of the thymus." It can increase the possibility of infections and autoimmune diseases.

The autoimmune system is a dynamic, ever-changing, ever-learning system. It develops from our early days and keeps developing until we take our last breath. The job of fighting of infections and invading pathogens takes years of preparation, training and relearning.

As I said earlier, experts believe that stress can make the thymus rescind earlier than usual due to an overstimulation of the parasympathetic fibers. This condition is infrequent and scarce but a more common issue is the early deactivation of the organ due to the overstimulation of the sympathetic fibers.

The thymus is a training center for the white blood cells. A fully functional thymus will continue to churn out fully trained and qualified white blood cells to police the body. When the thymus begins to decline for whatever reasons, it starts to affect the standards of white blood cells in the body. The white blood cells are not as qualified and educated as before and the standard of their protection begins to lag. This usually happens as we grow older and it explains why we are more susceptible to diseases and infections as we grow older. The white blood cells are losing their ability to protect the body, leaving us at the risk of attack. The attack doesn't only come from infections and invading pathogens but it can also come from the white blood cells themselves. The body's protectors (the white blood cells), will have lost some of their ability to distinguish between invaders and healthy body cells and they may end up attacking healthy cells in their quest to defend the body.

It manages the communication line between the immune system and the microbiome

Since our first discovery of the bacteria that reside in the human digestive tract, we have made significant leap in the past centuries discovering new information about the bacteria and their effect on the digestive system and the human body in general. The bacteria in our gut aid have numerous impacts on our health and examples of the sectors they affect include digestion and the nutrients available in ingested food, mood, brain functions and neurotransmitters. The total population of bacterial present in the gut is around 100 trillion. They are virtually the most populous residents of the human body and their contributions affect several aspect and functions of the body and its organs.

The vagus nerve serves as the line of communication between the microbiome and the other parts of the body. It is not alone in this task, as it enjoys support from hormones and the bloodstream. The gut and the activities of gut bacterial are also the most noticeable of the organs and systems involved with the vagus nerve. Take carvings for example, carving a certain food is our most basic interaction with the gut. It is a message from the bacterial of the gut informing you about their nutritional needs. Examples of gut bacteria are Bifidobacterium (a.k.a. Bifido) and Lactobacillus (a.k.a. Lacto). The knowledge that food cravings are signals transmitted by gut bacteria through the vagus nerve allows you to take charge of your diet. You can take back control and decide on dietary choices that will benefit the gut bacterial and the entire body instead of what the bacteria craves.

It allows us to create new memories

The scientific world has known for a while that the bacteria in the gut contribute to the development of the enteric nervous system but a more recent discovery has disclosed that gut bacteria also contribute to the central nervous system. When the vagus nerve transmit information between gut bacteria and the brain, it is possible that this line of communication is responsible for the secretion of Brain-Derived Neurotrophic Factor (BDNF). Brain-derived neurotrophic factor is a protein that increases neuronal connectivity and the ability of the brain to produce new memories.

This denotes that gut bacteria and the vagus nerve influence neuronal connectivity and the ability of the brain to produce new memories. If both function properly then there is the possibility of improving the brain and a reverses can also impair brain activity. This means that we can manipulate the neuronal connectivity and the ability to create new memories through the vagus nerve and gut bacteria.

The human body starts developing barriers and defense mechanism to protect itself from external threat from the fetal stage. One of such barriers is the blood barrier, it is our protection against invading bacteria, both good and bad. It is made up of the same cell as the blood-brain barrier. They are both susceptible to the same conditions and inflammation.

One of the most common effects of brain inflammation is brain fog. It is one of those moments when a person can't remember an essential word or the place they are. This is due to a temporary slip in the blood-brain barrier, which allows signals of inflammation to enter the brain and distort the functionality of neurons.

SECTION TWO

Chapter three: How does the vagus nerve work?

Chapter four: What can go wrong with the vagus nerve?

HOW DOES THE VAGUS NERVE WORK?

Like i said in the first chapter, neurons are the basic units that make up the vagus nerve. They transmit signals between cells and organs of the body. These signals may information or instructions, afferent or efferent signals.

Sending signals in neurons

Only 20% of the signals sent through the vagus nerve are efferent, the remaining 80% are afferent signals. Efferent signals are like information about the state of the union, about the conditions of the body organs, if the situation remains constant or changes. The vagus nerve is the largest communication system in the body. It reaches extend to the gut, immune system, the liver, pancreas, the brain and various other organs. The dendrites and long axons of the neuron cells are used to transmit the signals. The distances that most of these signals have to travel are long, so they have to be insulated so that the signal can arrive at its destination. The consequences of the signals not reaching their destination can bear disastrous consequences for the body.

Fat acts as insulators for these electrical signals. The cells of the human body store fat and the fat insulates and influences the transmission of these signals. The vagus nerve is protected by the same cells that protect all the other nerves of the body, the Schwann cells. The Schwann cells produce myelin sheath, which acts insulating barriers that ensures optimal functionality of the nerves and the protection of signals. Imagine the signals as an electric signal and the Schwann cells as the insulators that ensure that the signals remain within the chords or in our situation the neurons. If the Schwann cells malfunction or get compromised, the insulation is affected and the signal will be lost before it reaches its intended destination.

The body and its Schwann cells begin to produce myelin sheath when we are still fetuses, from at least 24 weeks in the mother's womb. The production of myelin sheath continues to increase until around our 40th week in mother's womb, by then we have reached full term. From the period henceforth the production of myelin sheath remains constant or varies slightly until we attain adolescent, after which it starts to recede.

Neurotransmitters

The neuron is like a cable and when the signal reaches the other end of that neuron it creates a neurotransmitter by producing a charge and releasing into the destination cell. The end of a neuron is called the terminal axon. Although there are several neurotransmitters present in the body, the vagus nerve almost exclusive uses the Acetylcholine (ACh). Two different structures combine to ACh, these two are choline and acetyl coenzyme A (acetyl-CoA). Free fatty acid and glucose are metabolized to form acetyl coenzyme A.

These metabolic processes are very specific and they require certain micronutrients.

The metabolism of glucose requires the following micronutrients in large quantity including chromium, coenzyme Q10, vitamin B1, lipoic acid and vitamin B3. The metabolism of free fatty acid on the other hand requires vitamin B2 and carnitine. The problem is the body doesn't have these micronutrients in sufficient supply.

Choline on the other hand is a vital micronutrient for animals. It cannot be produced by the body but it can be found in amino acids. Proteins such as soy, beef, turkey liver, chicken and egg yolks have the highest supply of choline. It can also be found in soy lecithin which is used as an additive in some processed foods.

Choline and acetyl coenzyme combine together in the neurons to form ACh. The ACh is then released into the cell or organ through the vagus neuron axons. This is how the neurotransmitter relaying the signal is transferred to the destination cell or organ.

The importance of choline and acetyl coenzyme to this process cannot be overstated. That is why we need to ensure that the body has adequate supply of both.

The actions of the signal in the destination organ

The neurotransmitter is not released directly into the destination cell or organ. It is instead released into a small space between the neurotransmitter and the cell, called a synapse. Large quantities of the neurotransmitter are released into the synapse. They then located receptor proteins of the cell that they can attach to.

Since we are talking about the vagus nerve, let's be more specific and talk about its major neurotransmitter, ACh. ACh binds itself to receptor proteins on the surface of cells after it is released into the synapse. These receptors are usually muscarinic acetylcholine receptors (mAChR), which are actually slow receptors or the much faster nicotinic acetylcholine receptors (nAChR).

Each AChR has its own type of receptor that receives signals from it and induces the required reaction in the cell. Neuron cells use muscarinic versions, while non-neuron cells and most organs use the nicotinic receptor.

The quantity of available receptor protein can be influenced by several factors. Take the activities of some gut bacteria which release LPS into the intestine and disrupt the production of receptor proteins. LPS reduces the activity of the genes that are responsible for the creation of receptor proteins.

WHAT CAN GO WRONG WITH THE VAGUS NERVE?

The body and the mind

The body and the mind have unquestionable power over each other. Why the body is unhealthy, the mind will also be unhealthy and when the mind is unhealthy the body will be unhealthy. An unhealthy body also equals an unhealthy mind, this saying can also be reversed to an unhealthy mind equals an unhealthy body. In the later decades of the last century, medical doctors and health practitioner crossed a new line in health studies. They discovered health problems caused to the body by the mind. The term for this is psychosomatics or psychosomatic medicine. The study of how psychological and social factors can affect the health.

Psychology today is much different from the psychoanalysis movement started by Sigmund Freud and his contemporaries. Psychoanalysis used to take years before the patient can attain a breakthrough significant enough to be release from therapy. While psychoanalysis still takes years for some patients, the modern world has reduced the average timeline of therapy. It saves time and cost, since therapy sessions are usually expensive. To make psychoanalysis more effective than or at least as effective as it used to be we have moved to a reliance on pills and prescription drugs.

The patient still relies on the prescription drugs after leaving therapy. The prescription drugs are also expensive but they are not as expensive as an average therapy session.

Don't get me wrong because I am not trying to condemn modern psychology and psychiatry. They do work, but it doesn't usually offer long term solution and it is still considerably expensive. It may also have some side effects on other aspects of the patient's health and behavior. Over time the patient may also become desensitized to the drug and it will become ineffective. Then the process of finding another viable prescription drug and a functional dosage plan comes back again.

There are other avenues to modern medicine that we are not exploiting.

This chapter is about health problems that can be attributed to the vagus nerve and can therefore be treated by stimulating the vagus nerve.

Some of these health problems may be psychological as expressed above but physical problems are the most common. Most of these health problems are related to the nervous system, which means they can be treated by stimulating the vagus nerve. They may also be related to our ability to manage stress and control our emotions.

Fear and anxiety

Anxiety has always been one of the major focuses of psychology and psychoanalysis. It still retains its position today. Everyone gets anxious, it is a vital part of our humanity. We can see it as a flaw or as a blessing. It can help us make the right decision because we will know a decision or task is important when we feel anxious. Anxiety should however be temporary and if we start to feel it compulsively over a long period of time, then it becomes a problem. It affects our daily life and ability to function. Anxiety can be crippling and every time you think you have hit the bottom, down you sink again. That's the big problem with anxiety, there is barely any hope that it will get better but you know that it can get worse and it definitely will. Anxiety is not a rare problem suffered by only a fraction of the population as most people like to think. In the united states alone, over 18 percent of the population is suffers from anxiety at one point in their lives.

Anxiety is born out of fear. It can even be described as constant, crippling fear. Fear itself is a product of the nervous system. The central nervous system secretes the chemicals that become fear when faced with a threat. It is a reaction of the sympathetic nerves stimulated through the dorsal branch of the vagus nerve. Anxiety is being under constant stress which puts the body in a perpetual fight or flight situation, with a lot of emphasis on flight.

It manifest itself physically by altering the breathing pattern to raise the heart rate, releasing stress hormones, inability to communicate properly and excessive sweating among others. All of these can be used to describe anxiety but there is one major difference between fear and anxiety. Fear is generated by a current and viable threat while anxiety is not. The threat in anxiety is born out of the imagination. It doesn't really exit, at least not in the manner that anxiety projects it. Anxiety may wander to our memories and dredge out a threat from the past or travel to the future to generate an imaginary and monstrous threat. It doesn't matter where the threat comes from or how it looks and feels like. The point is that it is not real, it is only a figment of the imagination.

When the threat responsible for anxiety attack is actually real, we become guilty of exaggerating it.

Anxiety can become extreme with panic attacks and phobias.

Panic attack is a brief and intense experience of terror and anxiety. It comes with a bang, fast and furious and it usually leaves in less than ten minutes. The feeling lingers for a while after the attack. There are several factors that can trigger and anxiety attack. Most of these generates stress on the mind, enough stress to finally snap the mind.

Physical manifestations of anxiety attacks are similar to those of fear but multiply to a thousand folds. The body gives way and begins to tremble, it shakes and starts sweating profusely. The mind becomes distorted and dizzy.

The only way to fight anxiety is to bring the body out of it constant state of fight or flight. Various exercises that stimulate the vagus nerve can be used to accomplish this. Recovery from anxiety is a regular process that operates on setting long term goals.

Phobias are the most common types of anxiety. Just a little less than 12 percent of the world's population suffers from one form of phobia. Some people even have multiple phobias. It is that extreme fear focused on something. That focal object of the fear becomes the trigger. It may be an event, activity, living or non-living object. Like all forms of anxiety, it is due to the stimulation of the sympathetic nerves of the central nervous system.

One of the problems with phobia is the constant anticipation of encountering the focal object of the phobia. It can seem wore than the encounter itself. You can't really sole it because there is no logical explanation for the overwhelming fear. When treating phobia with psychoanalysis, most techniques focus on the focal object of fear and the root of the fear. Therefore they tend to find biological and early developmental reasons for phobia and other form of anxiety.

Some phobias may be seen so strange and unbelievable but you must understand that the fear must have been viable when it starting. The mind just didn't grow to overcome that fear.

You need to understand a phobia before you can confront and heal it. There are numerous sources online that provide information on different phobias and their treatment. Wikipedia provides a list of all know phobias. You can start there for a general overview, and then search more reliable sources once you know what you are looking for.

Inability to breath properly

Most health problems associated with the vagus nerve usually have dysfunctional breathing as one of their symptoms. This is because breathing is one of the most obvious functions associated to the vagus nerve, making it one of the most first insight into the condition of the vagus nerve.

Breathing is the first thing we learn to do at birth. Most of our organs are already working in the womb, but mother is breathing on our behalf when we are in the womb. The moment we come into the world we must immediately start breathing. We wouldn't survive our first few seconds without breathing.

We have help, the midwife or doctor may clear the airway to allow air into the lungs. The main task falls to the central nervous system and the diaphragm. The diaphragm also needs help from the lungs which are signaled to open or close by the vagus nerve.

Our body learns to breathe properly as a baby, through the diaphragm. We are using the major muscles to breathe instead of the accessory muscles.

As we grow up, the body may forget how to breathe through the diaphragm. This may be due to stress and other social factors. Proper breathing requires the belly to move, protruding in and out, this clashes with some cultural values.

Some aspects of psychology believe that we copy other people's mannerisms and try to fit into society's idea of who we should be because we started out in a position of inferiority. When we are born into the world, we are at the mercy of our parents, guardians and other adults. We worship them and we want to be like them. That is how we grow and learn. We learn to work by mimicking older people, we learn to speak by trying to remake the sounds that comes out of their mouth. This process applies to several aspects of our life as we grow up. Even as adults we still, mimic others.

Like is said earlier, breathing through the diaphragm moves the abdomen a lot. This makes the person appear to have a big belly and look fat. Sure, a mildly protruding stomach doesn't technically make you fat, but our society has its standard of beauty.

That standard prioritizes a thin and flat stomach.

In trying to fit into society's image of beauty, why try to hide the belly and this affects breathing. This later becomes second nature to us that the body becomes used to it. It begins to breathe improperly.

Repetitive hiding of the stomach may work and it wills seem like we are training the stomach muscles to maintain a shape but we are actually training the nerves that signals the muscles.

The increase of blood flow to the muscles allows it to grow. Since we trained the nerves to breath improperly we can also reteach it to breathe properly.

A nerve and muscle has to function often or it will become slow and dysfunctional.

For superficial reasons, we have trained the body to breathe inefficiently and improperly from our teenage years and this has become second nature, ingrained into the fibers of our being. It affects the nerves that have not been utilized properly for so long. The phrenic nerves are not being properly utilized, the nerve that signal the lungs, the vagus nerve is also not being utilized properly.

We can get back on the healthy breathing pattern but that is a topic for the next chapter, so make sure you finish this book. If you want to know the importance of breathing properly, you don't have to look further than the various therapy and other healing techniques that utilize different breathing techniques.

Inability to maintain a normal heart rate

The resting heart rate depends on how healthy, calm and confident we are. The average heart rate is supposed to be between 60 to 100bpm. A healthier heart rate may be as low as 50bpm while anything more than 100bpm can be disastrous to the health. The sympathetic nerves and the vagus nerve will dictate a change the heat rate. The sympathetic nerves will try to increase the heart rate but the vagus nerves will try to keep it a slow as it can. A considerably low heart rate, especially under stress implies that the vagus nerve is strong and functioning optimally. A strong vagus nerve can also increase the lifespan. Some research show that a low heart rate can result in longer life. A well-functioning vagus nerve keeps the heart rate low, which means that it can expand your lifespan.

A dysfunctional heart rate is due to the inability of the vagus nerve to reduce it after the body encounters stress.

It takes the heart a few minutes to return to its resting value. This return to resting heart rate from a high heart rate after the stressors have activated the sympathetic muscles is called recovery. The amount of time it takes the body to recover depends on the vagus nerve. A strong vagus nerve allows you to quickly calm your nerves and slow down your heart rate. The opposite happens with a dysfunctional heart rate.

There is also the problem of the vagus nerve over functioning and the sympathetic nerves under functioning. The job is split into two in order to maintain balance. The job of the parasympathetic nerves is to slow down the heart rate, while that of the sympathetic nerve is to quicken the heart rate. If the parasympathetic nerves are functioning more than the parasympathetic nerves, the heart rate will be too low due to an imbalance in the nervous system and it can result in fainting, which is a temporary loss of consciousness. The medical term for fainting is called syncope. Fainting may not be directly life threatening, but it is inconvenient at best. It can affect the ability to function properly. It can also be embarrassing, if it happens at inconvenient times in public gatherings.

The person doesn't have to be sick or have an existing health condition. Syncope can occur in an otherwise healthy individual. Again, it doesn't have any long-term effect, neither is it life threatening but it can have a devastating effect on the mood and self-confidence.

Many people believe that a sudden physical head tilt can cause this imbalance. This includes motions like standing or sitting too fast after lying down for a long period of time. The sudden shift in posture results in the direction of blood flow and blood pooling location. The change is too sudden for the muscles of the heart to easy adjust to. In our theoretical scenario, the blood pool location moves to the abdominal region from the chest area. This results in a change in blood pressure, reducing it significantly and thus triggering the episode. It is the job of the autonomic nerves to maintain blood pressure and they have failed in the task. They try to regain control and the person starts regaining consciousness when they do. The episode leaves the body drained, fatigued and nauseated.

This example discusses the trigger for the fainting spell but it doesn't talk about why the autonomous nervous system wasn't able to perform its duty properly during the change in posture. It was unable to regulate the blood vessels and the muscles of the heart properly enough to accommodate the aforementioned action. This reduction in the ability of the autonomous nervous system to regulate the nerves is called dysautonomia. Dysautonomia may be a hereditary disease. It can also be due to other non-hereditary diseases such as Ehlers-Danlos syndrome and Charcot-Marie-Tooth disease. It may also be a physical manifestation of other issues related to the digestive and autoimmune system such as chiari malfunctions, physical trauma, surgery or pregnancy.

It may be due to lack of some nutrients required by the components of the nervous system or due to increasing level of toxins in the body. Conditions like these are due to the inability of the nerves to react quickly.

Dysfunctional breathing can also directly affect the nerves of the autonomous system and the organs that are innervated by them. Examples of these diseases are chronic neural inflammation, ulcerative colitis, sarcoidosis, Sjogren's syndrome, Crohn's disease, Parkinson's disease and amyloidosis.

The severity of vasovagal syncope is different for people dealing with it. The condition may be mild or severe. You need to understand that vasovagal syncope is not a disease in itself. It is instead a symptom of another problem. A person experiencing fainting spells should visit the doctor. Neurological tests such as MRI scan will probably be required. You may find out the problem but sometimes vasovagal syncope is just a consequence of an improperly functioning autonomous nervous system, to be more specific, an overactive vagus nerve and an underactive sympathetic nerve.

When the body doesn't seem to be able to properly regulate the blood pressure and heart rate, this is usually the problem.

Chronic stress

The sympathetic nerves are in charge of handling stress. As stress increases on the body, and the body maintains its fight or flight mode, the body increases its ability to deal with the stress. The power of the sympathetic nerves increase with the increase in stress levels, blood is pumped to the hands and leg in order to better handle the stress. The body secretes chemicals such as adrenaline in order to handle the stress.

The stress may get to a point that the body can't take it anymore. It becomes unable to increase its stressor levels. It has reached the limit.

Stress can be good for us, consider the beginning. The body improved itself to meet the stress, it was only until later that it couldn't handle it anymore. The good kind of stress as the stress that makes us grow is called has a technical name. This technical name is "eustress." Eustress is helps us to grow and improve our self. It helps us to expand our horizons and conquer new territories. Examples of eustress include competition, relationships, taking on new challenges and working out.

Events do occur that add the negative kind of stress. This kind of stress is technically called "distress." Examples of distress include health problems, relationship problems, career problems and financial problems.

The body senses them as negative stress, unnecessary additional weigh on the shoulder. The difference lies in perception and the effect the stress has on the body.

These two kinds of stresses move us in different direction. Eustress or negative stress builds us up while negative stress pulls us down.

While some stress fit conveniently into either of the two types, perception is still king. It is what you believe the stress to be that gives it power over you. Take the loss of a good paying job as an example. This kind of stressor should easily fit into the distress category (negative stress), but your view and perception of it can propel it into eustress. You can see it as a blessing in disguise and it won't have too much negative effect on you. Let's use another example of a mild inconvenience such as having to trek a few distance in order to get some groceries because the nearby grocery store was closed.

Let's say the distance is not far, so you decided to go on foot. This shouldn't be an issue unless you make it into one. Instead of approaching it with a negative attitude and turning it into a stressful event, try to approach it as an opportunity to exercise and stretch your legs. Enjoy the scenery on your way.

These two examples are just simple analogies, the real world will be more complicated. You won't be aware of all the factors contributing to the stresses in your daily life.

Some stresses may be hidden by other more immediate and noticeable stresses. Most of the major internal stresses in our lives are due to habit and lifestyle. Once you can identify these harmful habits then it becomes possible to change them. Changing livelong habits won't be easy, it is definitely harder than recognizing the habits themselves, which can sometimes be harder than we expect. But recognizing the habit is just the first step. It is also not enough to just recognize them. I repeat, you need to make conscious daily efforts for change.

The body itself has the same reaction to every stressor. It doesn't matter if it is eustress or distress, they are perceived the same way. We automatically switch into fight or flight mode. This mode ensures quick decision making and quick action. It is still the same two options in the mode, fight or flight.

The body shifts from the comfort of the rest or digest mode. It reduces the flow of blood to the various organs in favor of sending them to the legs and arms.

The relationship between the fight or flight mode and the rest or digest mode is not binary. It is not one or the other. It is actually a circle, a continuum between the two modes. The modes are at extreme ends of the continuum, like the 6'O Clock and 12'O Clock positions on an analogue clock or the endpoints of a single line. Both of these examples work. The spaces between them are a variation of either of the two modes.

The body functions optimally in the parasympathetic side of the scales. The parasympathetic side is the rest or digest side of the continuum. The human body should spend about 80 percent of its time in the rest or digest side. We can't do that without a fully functional vagus nerve. When we do activate the vagus nerve and stay on the rest or digest side, it means that the body can handle the stress currently thrown at it and stimulate the sympathetic nerves to accommodate more stress.

We must also note how easy it is to move from the rest or digest mode (parasympathetic) into the fight or flight mode (sympathetic). It can happen in a fraction of a second, the body can send signals over long distances very quickly through the hormone cortisol and the neurotransmitter adrenalin. There is no boot period and the body can switch from one end of the spectrum to the other quickly, but it is much faster and easier to move towards the fight or flight mode.

Imagine the rest and digest mode as lying down in the tranquility of a private beach, enjoying the view with no one around. Then someone enters this personal and private time. Either the person maintains a distance or not, he has entered your personal space and disrupted the serenity of the environment. Now imagine how annoying it would be if the person actually started displaying obnoxious behavior or trying to talk to you when you are not interested in having a conversation. At any point in this analogy, the parasympathetic nerves would have kicked in and you will be in the fight or flight mode. Even if or when the person leaves, you are still going to be stressed and it will take some time before you return to the rest or digest mode, if you can.

The analogy explains the process of shifting between the two modes. It shows how easy it is to enter the fight or flight mode and how slightly harder it is to switch to the rest or digest mode.

It may be trickier and easier to stay in the fight or flight mode, but that is where the problem begins. Remaining in the fight or flight mode case a state of perpetual stress that is known as chronic stress. It leaves the body unable to manage more stress.

The body may remain in fight or flight mode just because it already spends most of its time in the mode. It is always under stress that it becomes tired of switching to fight or flight mode, then return to rest or digest mode, only to go back to fight or flight mode not long after, because the body is always in constant stress.

Remember that your perception of stress also factor in because it determines if the body will interpret the stress as negative stress or positive stress.

Ultimately, remaining in the fight or flight mode reduces the activity of the vagus nerve, since that is its job, to take the body out of the fight or flight mode. The vagus nerve begins to slow down and becomes rusty (permit me to use that word) like a retired athlete. The sympathetic nerves are the ones in control, because the body remains in their zone.

Any added stress big or small adds to the burden until it becomes chronic. The champion vagus nerve that is supposed to return the body to rest or digest mode can't even do that in a minor stress incident because it has already been conquered by the bigger stressor. Let's use an analogy of the AIDS. Don't mind me but I believe it fits properly into this situation. AIDS destroys the white blood cells and antibodies, ultimately reducing the body's ability to defend itself. Due to the reduced defensive capabilities of the body or lack of it entirely, minor health issues begin to seriously harass the body.

I believe that the vagus nerve is similar to the body in our analogy. It can't manage the small stresses again because the small stresses are literally riding on the back of bigger stresses that have incapacitated the vagus nerve.

A fellow road user cuts you off, you should definitely get angry but the anger has to subsidize. For someone with a dysfunctional vagus nerve the anger may become road rage. Sure he is angry at the road user but is the event worth the emotional effort.

That is what chronic stress does to you. It impairs your ability to activate the vagus nerve and manage smaller stress. The longer chronic stress remains the more it incapacitates the parasympathetic nerves of the vagus nerve.

It effects go beyond emotional management issues. It impairs other bodily functions that involve the vagus nerve. These include effects on the digestive system, the entire autoimmune system, detoxification of the body, inflammation and so on.

It results in multiple health conditions in one person because numerous organs are involved. As said earlier it is easy to make changes. Prescription drugs and medications will only treat the symptoms which appear to be the disease. The disease is a dysfunction of the vagus nerves and fixing it will make it easier for the body to recover from the many associated problems.

A dysfunctional vagus nerve is treatable as I sated earlier. You need to reduce your stress levels which involve changing some habits and making new lifestyle choices.

The good thing is that patients who make these changes have seen swift and significant recovery.

Many exercise to help you stay in the in the rest or digest mode will be explored in the next chapter.

Stress management test

The inability to handle stressful situations is one of the biggest issues with a dysfunctional vagus nerve. The modern world is filed with stressors, so you can't stay away from it. People who can't handle stress are always overwhelmed with emotions. This is due to the inability of the vestibular canals to suppress the emotions. These vestibular canals are connected to the autonomic nervous system. The situation denotes an imbalance in the autonomic nervous system. The parasympathetic nerves are too powerful for the sympathetic nerves so they end up overpowering them. In order to test how compromised the vagus nerve is, you can try the spinning chair test. Sit in a spin chair and spin the chair while keeping your eyes open. The idea is to monitor your heart rate and the body's reaction to the exercise. The exercise is similar to the head tilt example used in "inability to maintain a normal heart rate. You can also use the head tilt exercise to test your ability to measure stress.

Chronic inflammation

When the vagus nerve is not functioning properly, one of the first hints is the inability of the body to properly manage inflammation. It means the vagus nerve is not effectively doing its job, which is to act as a message network between the immune system and the brain. There are many factors that can cause inflammation. That is why experts rarely look at the vagus nerve.

Inflammation can be corrected only when we find out what was responsible for it.

Inflammation may be mild and we know that inflammation is the body's way of defending itself. Inflammation really becomes a health problem when it becomes chronic.

Chronic inflammation can manifest itself physically in many ways, from cancer, to auto immune diseases, growth of tumor, and arthritis etc.

Inflammation becomes chronic due to the inability of the vagus nerve to transmit the signals required to stop inflammation. You can try to stimulate the vagus nerve and improve the vagal tone. This improves the vagus nerve's ability to transmit signals between the white blood cells and the brain. Effective signaling from the vagus nerve will reverse inflammation without need for any medication. Then the body can try to repair the damaged cells.

Some of the most common inflammation is caused by physical and emotional trauma so

I would like to discuss the relationship between these kinds of inflammation and the vagus nerve. I will also discuss the two main inflammation issues caused by the dysfunctions of the vagus nerve. These are chronic inflammation of the gut and autoimmune conditions.

Inflammation caused by physical and emotional trauma

Physical traumas cause the most obvious types of inflammation. When you sprain an ankle or bump a body part, it soon becomes red, swollen and sore. This is due to the actions of the white blood cells. The cells increase blood flow and secretion to chemicals to the spot in order to repair the damage and fight any invading pathogen. These symptoms are only supposed to exist for a short period of time pending the time that the body heals itself. When they remain it starts to harm the body. It means the cholinergic anti-inflammatory pathway (which acts as a signal network between the antibodies) and the vagus nerve has failed in their task of transmitting information.

There are various reasons for inflammation to remain over a longer than normal period of time. All these reasons prevent the body from healing properly.

One curve ball responsible for inflammation is emotional trauma. This stress applied on the mind can create a negative attitude that affects one's perception of the environment and other people. Emotional trauma may vary in severity and the impact on the individual. The impact of emotional trauma can also be affected by the number of emotionally traumatic event and the how closely together they happen. It is easier for us to recover from things that happened few years apart than for something that happened a few days apart.

Emotionally traumatic events trigger the sympathetic forces that put us in fight or flight mode. This increases the likeliness of inflammation and reduces the ability of the vagus nerve to stop inflammation.

Emotional trauma rarely acts alone. It combines with physical trauma (the quick and ready cause of inflammation) to form a deadly combination. Any inflammation from physical trauma is expanded by the actions of the emotional trauma.

In the end, inflammation becomes chronic and more complicated health problem start to rear their heads. Much like the way chronic stress works, small physical trauma can lead to more complicated health problems, because numerous other emotional and physical trauma have complicated the parasympathetic nerves of the vagus nerve.

Chronic Inflammation of the Gut

The white blood cells can become desensitized to inflammation, if inflammation occurs constantly over a long period of time. These white blood cells are the little soldiers of the body. They protect it. Constant inflammation will impact them negatively.

Inflammation in the gut is a tricky situation because we can't easily identify the symptoms. It doesn't manifest externally until the situation becomes really severe. You can find a test online or visit your health provider.

An imbalance in the microbiome population of the digestive tract is the most common factor responsible for inflammation in the gut. There are other causes such as the consumption of inflammatory food items but the aforementioned one is the most rampant one.

It is not just the white blood cells and antibodies that can get desensitized to inflammation. Constant inflammation can also wear out the vagus nerve. It begins to learn to ignore inflammatory signals which results in a disastrous situation because it ignores its job which is to send signals to the antibodies to stop inflammation. When it doesn't do its job, the inflammation won't stop and the antibodies will start to attack healthy cells of the body.

Young people are relatively safe, but inflammation begins to get worse after you reach 30 years of age. The functionality of vagus nerve and vagal tone has reduced significantly. It has learned over the years to ignore inflammatory symptoms and signals. It not just age that reduces the influence of the vagus nerve and vagal tone on inflammation, other situations that put people in delicate health conditions can also cause it. Examples include, pregnancy and childbirth, sickness and emotional trauma.

Autoimmune Conditions

Chronic stress, our lifestyle and poor dietary choices contribute to autoimmune conditions. It is one of the most rapidly growing health conditions in the United States. Examples of autoimmune health conditions include heumatoid arthritis, alopecia areata, Graves' disease, Hashimoto's thyroiditis, psoriasis, multiple sclerosis, Crohn's disease, systemic lupus erythematosus, type 1 diabetes and celiac disease, and many others. There are much more where that came from.

Most of these health conditions start in the digestive tract, which is fitting because the digestive tract contains the single largest population of immune cells. These cells are located here in large quantities because it is also the point of access into the body for many toxinx, pathogens and chemicals. The other point of access is broken skin but it is not nearly as porous as the mouth and digestive tract.

The immune cells are lined along the walls of the digestive tract. They are held in lymphatic tissues built like pocket spaces called GALT. You can visit the second chapter for more information.

The immune cells of the digestive tract encounter numerous invaders which they are there to fight against. Persistent entrance of these invading toxins and pathogens can desensitize the immune cells to them. Over a long period of time, they begin to stop reacting to and fighting the invaders. They have worked so hard that have become third. This is how autoimmune problems start.

Some autoimmune diseases are hereditary, but it still requires to be triggered. According to a Hartmut Wekerle in a review published in Rheumatology in 2016, the following three factors contribute to the risk of developing an autoimmune disease. Here they are:

- An amount of autoimmune, autoreactive T cells in the GALT

- An imbalance in the gut microbiome that is pro-inflammation

- Hereditary genes that are susceptible to autoimmune conditions

There isn't much we can do about the first and last factors. We don't know the amount of autoimmune cells in the GALT, we also can't change our genes. What we can do is to influence the second factor, the balance of microbiome in the gut. We can do this by feeding the microbiome with the right food items.

Post-Traumatic Stress Disorder (PTSD)

Post-traumatic stress disorder (PTSD) first came to public attention after World War 1, then it was called shell shock and the public was divided over it. There is barely any division over the legality of PTSD as a medical condition today, which is a good thing, the bad part is that PTSD has become more common in our society. Many people today are suffering from PTSD, far more than you would think because most people expect only soldiers and armed combatants to be suffering from PTSD, but anyone who has been subjected to a traumatic event can suffer from PTSD.

The autonomic nervous system and trauma

The autonomic nervous system is very resilient and can easily recover from many events. Some people are more resilient than others. There are some traumatic events that can be too severe for the autonomic nervous system to handle and it will be unable recover unaided.

We all have our own specific reaction to a traumatic event. No matter how shocking the event is some people feel all they need to feel and express all they need to express. After that, they can move on as their autonomic nervous system recovers from the shock and intensity of the event. The recovery may not be quick or easy but it is moderate for the average person and faster than some people.

Some people may not be that lucky. They remain in that moment, dwelling in it and reliving it form that day henceforth. Their illusion of reality has been chattered and they are forever changed by the event, not in a good way. The event keeps draining and affecting them long after it happened. This is a state of perpetual fight or flight mode.

The sympathetic nerves are activated after a traumatic event but the parasympathetic nerves are unable to return the body to rest or digest mode. This doesn't mean that they have PTSD. It means that they "could" have

PTSD or depression. The activation of the sympathetic nerves may lead to a perpetual fight or flight response. That is what causes PTSD. The sympathetic nerves could also lead to a withdrawal or shutdown response, which is depression. Depression puts the autonomous nervous system in chronic dorsal vagal mode.

These two are the major extreme reactions that the body has to trauma. Both reactions prevent the patient from properly integrating with society and mingling with friends and family. A person suffering from PTSD is also likely to exhibit symptoms of depression. It shows that PTSD is more complex and serious than depression. The inability to interact with society leaves many people with PTSD lonely and isolated. They may become violent or suicidal. we are yet to find a proper solution to PTSD. The options out there include medication and therapy but they are mostly designed to manage the situation.

Like I always say, you can't tackle a problem if you don't know the cause. Most people don't really talk about or understand the causes of PTSD. They know it is a reaction to a traumatic event, an event that happened in the past and the patient is still relieving it. They know that every spell is triggered by memories of the traumatic event and the patient relieves them whenever the spell occurs.

Most people don't consider it for what PTSD is, it is a twist of the reactions generated sympathetic by the sympathetic nerves (the fight or flight mode). Normal stress moves the autonomous nervous system towards the fight or flight mode. PTSD is actually a chronic dorsal vagal mode. The autonomic nervous system moves the body to hopelessness, fear and apathy, instead of fight or fear. This means you can't treat PTSD the same way you would treat other reactions of the sympathetic nerves such as chronic stress. It would be counter-productive and it may elevate the conditions of the patient.

Psychologist and other medical practitioners often focus on the traumatic event when treating PTSD. They don't usually study the Patients psychological fixation on the traumatic event. It is the memories that trigger a spell. Telling someone, (definitely a professional) about the event may alleviate the impact of the condition. It could also backfire by triggering an episode. Recalling an intense event may send the person into a hypnotic trance. It stimulates the emotions and brings back the even with vivid details.

The psychologist may try other techniques such as integrating different techniques and exercises in treating a patient and helping the patient integrate back into society.

PTSD and the dorsal branch

One of the best ways to treat PTSD is to target the dorsal branch state. Bring the patient out of that mode and all may be well. This procedure is a gradual process that needs to be practiced until it becomes second nature.

The dorsal vagal mode is not just a psychological issue, it is much more than that. The problem won't be solved by talk therapy alone. It is more a combination of a physical and psychological issue. That is why it is aptly called a psychophysiological issue. The treatment of these kinds of health conditions with medication and drugs such as antidepressants and other stimulants only arouses the autonomous nervous system. It triggers the patient to be optimistic by releasing feel good chemicals into the bloodstream but it doesn't solve the main issue, which is why drugs alone are not the answer. It doesn't make the patient want to reintegrate into society or feel true happiness and joy.

Understanding the relationship between the dorsal branches of the vagus nerve and its relationship with PTSD can help in the treatment of the disorder. It will help in the treatment of other psychophysiological disorders and also psychological disorders. The dorsal branches activities on the visceral organs caused PTSD. It is a state that decreases the ability of a patient and their love ones to live their live effectively and happily. The treatments we have today are very expensive and not exactly efficient. It is an improvement on the way PTSD used to be treated in the past but we still have a long way to go before we can get it right. The next step in the journey involves the vagus nerve. It involves properly examining the relationship between the autonomous nervous system and PTSD and using our understanding of that relationship to treat the disorder. Why medications and pills have not been the answer it may be possible to bring a person suffering from PTSD to fully functional recovery and social integration through the manipulation of the autonomic nervous system, where the problem really is.

The autonomic nervous system and depression

The population of the American public dealing with depression is baffling. Depression is now worse than obesity. Out of all the mental health conditions in the United

States, about 10 percent is depression. American has turned to prescription churning out pills and handing them out to pretty much any of these depressed people. Antidepressants and related medications are the most prescribed and purchased medications. They account for a third of all the prescription drugs used in the United States. This problem is not just an American issue. The sales of antidepressants in 2013 raked in north of $9.8 billion.

The most obvious symptom of depression is the lack of interest. A person battling depression doesn't want to do anything, especially with other people. They are apathetic, inactive, unmotivated, lack appetite or eat too much and many other.

Depression is about feelings, negative feelings. The negative feelings influence the person with depression's actions and habits. These are examples of the feelings that a depressed person has:

1. Sadness

2. Hopelessness

3. Emptiness

4. Shame

5. Guilt

6. Restlessness

7. Anxiety

8. Apathy

9. Lethargy

10. Lack of motivation

All of these emotions affect their memory and decision making ability. They are unable to concentrate and they may also experience pains and aches. Depression becomes extreme when the person starts self-harming or become suicidal. This is due to the activities of the sympathetic nerves which stimulate the autonomic nervous system into a chronic dorsal mode.

A medical caregiver such as a therapist or doctor will question you and monitor your reactions and responses, even your medical history before than can diagnose you as a depressant. The doctor won't consider that the situation is a state, he believes is a temporary phase and prescribes you some drugs. The medication works but it is temporary and you have to take another one when it wears off. Then this becomes a daily thing and you get on the medication, taking it every day for the next few weeks, months or even years.

It becomes a thing until you become desensitized to the medication and you have to try a stronger dosage or a different drug. Medication doesn't really solve the problem it just helps you maintain it.

When you are already on a meditation it is a terrible idea to stop taking a meditation without the consent of a physician, especially the physician who prescribed it, if you can find him. That's not to say you shouldn't stop taking a meditation if you find a better option or you feel it is working, it just mean you should seek an experts opinion before making the decision and receive advice on the best way to proceed. This is mostly due to withdrawal. Most medicines have a withdrawal effect on the body. When you have taken a medication for so long that your body is used to having it in your bloodstream, you need to wean the body away from that drug. If this is not done properly the body may react.

The journal of the American Medical Association published a report that showed that antidepressants may not actually work if the depression is mild. This has not slowed down the American population that still purchases almost 300 million antidepressant prescriptions per year.

If the general public is not reading these credible sources of information, surely the doctors are. Yet they still prescribe antidepressants for anyone with a mild case of depressants. Sure therapists still want you to undergo talk therapy but when you complain about depression to your doctor you are most likely to visit the pharmacy.

So why do doctors still prescribe antidepressants or why do intelligent people who have access to the right information still ask for antidepressants?

The problem is similar with their treatments of PTSD. Most people, including doctors don t fully understand the impact of the autonomous nervous system. It is the main issue in this case and you have to affect it before you can treat depression. But antidepressants don't work on the autonomous nervous system because it is resilient and flexible. Any effect will be temporary because it will later adjust itself.

Medicine doesn't really pay attention to the physiology of depression; most of the emphasis is on the physiology of chronic stress. Doctors don't focus on the dorsal branch activity of the vagus nerve and the autonomous nervous system.

That is where our study of the anatomy of the vagus nerve comes in. It exposes a new understanding of the central nervous system, on that most people didn't pay attention to before and few are only beginning to consider. It shows that there are safe, efficient alternatives to our current techniques and processes for treating some diseases.

Poor social interaction and communication

Human beings are social animals. One of our oldest and most important institutions, marriage is designed to do one thing and one thing alone, protect us from being alone. We don't just marry for procreation sake. We grow up in family and when we have to leave, we create another family in an endless circle of life and interaction.

Why are we so desperate to be with other people? Because interaction with other people is vital to our wellbeing and when I say interaction, I mean face to face action, not just the behind the scenes interactions of the modern world. If you want to prove my point, I suggest you try spending a few days or a week at home, alone and with minimal contact with other people. The first part of you that will be affected is your mood. Then it will start to affect other parts of your body including your health. Social interaction with other people stimulates the vagus nerve. Social interaction is good for the autonomous nervous system which means it is good for us. One of the most efficient and simplest punishments is solitary confinement. Parents use the mild version of it on their young ones. They ground them, take away their phones or tell them to go into their rooms. This punishment might seem easy and soft but it if far from it. It has been working for generations, that is why we keep using it. Consider a more extreme version of it, the one that actually bears the name "solitary confinement." It is used in prison to punish violent and unruly inmates. It involves locking the prisoner alone without human contact over a period of time. They don't starve the prisoner, the person that brings his food is the only human being he is in contact with. That person doesn't even acknowledge him. He does everything he needs to do in the confinement. It could also get worse the confinement could be a very small and dark place. This is as alone as it gets and one can only imagine what the prisoner has gone to of feels, when he is released back with the other inmates.

Heart rate variability which we will later use to measure the functionality of the vagus nerve and vagal tone, reduces without contact with other people. The person starts to exhibit symptoms of depression.

A study by Kok et al in the journal of *Biological Psychology*, by Kok et al., in 2010 proved the importance of vagal tone to mood. The study measured the vagal tone of the subjects at the beginning of their program and 9 weeks later. The study should that subjects with better vagal tone have more positivity, while subjects with lower vagal tone portray more negative attitudes.

There are more studies like these that show the relationship between feelings and the vagus nerve.

This shows that we can train the vagus nerve to improve our mood and generate more positive attitudes. It means that we need to be around other people for the sake of our mood, attitude and health. The inability to mingle and interact with other people shows a dysfunction in the vagus nerves and it can cause inflammation and other health problems related to the vagus nerve.

Dysfunctional sleep

The brain goes through five stages in a cycle, when we sleep. The first two stages are associated with the early 7 to 15 minutes of sleep. They are both states of light sleep. The next two stages, stage 3 and four are states of deep restorative sleep. The autonomous nervous system begins to control the body's restoration and repair. The body's heart rate variability increases as it begins to prepare the body for the next day. Some of the actions it undertakes are:

1. Repair of tissues and muscles

2. Growth and development,

3. Boosting immune system functions

4. Production of energy in preparation for the next day

Stage 5 is called the Rapid-Eye Movement (REM) stage. This stage sees the decrease of the heart rate variability. The vagus nerve has completed its job in the last stage and the parasympathetic nerves let up. The sympathetic nerves take control. The sympathetic nerves begin to wander the memories and dreams happen.

The time that these stages will fall into varies with age. For adults, stage 1 to 4 occurs early at night. They tend to occur in a repeated cycle. Stage 5, itself occurs later in our sleep. It is why we may be able to recollect our dreams when we wake up, because we just dreamt them recently, in the final stages of our sleep. Each of these stages don't just occur ones. Each one is repeated a few times. REM, stage 5 usually occurs about 5 to 6 times every night. So does stage 3 and 4.

Stage 3 and 4 acts as a training and working session for the vagus nerve. We are in deep sleep and the autonomous nervous system takes control. This period cats as a literal gym session for the vagus nerve. It prepares for the day ahead. Remember than training makes the vagus nerve better. But since the vagus nerve only trains in stage 3 and 4, it means that our body must attain that stage of sleep. That means having a good and deep night rest. If you don't get a good night rest your body won't be able to reach deep restorative sleep, which is the training ground of the vagus nerve.

So how do you get a good sleep? What is the minimum time period needed for a good night rest or sleep? These are the questions to ask.

Experts prescribed 8 hours of sleep very night. Most people have to be up in the morning to take care of their duties and head to work so they feel that they can't afford to sleep for 8 hours every night. You can. How about you get to bed early, instead of watching late night television

What about having your meals, snacks and drinks at least two hours before your sleep time, in order not to disturb your sleep.

The afferent fibers of the vagus nerve allow it to clock the quantity of food that is currently in your stomach, especially at night. It monitors and restricts the amount of food that you eat. It does this by controlling the expansion of the stomach, specifically how large the stomach can expand. It reduces the sensitivity of the stomach to expansion, hereby ensuring that it can hold less food and you will become satiated. The vagus nerve does this at night that is why we mostly consume less food at night.

Dysfunctional liver

The liver is on of the most complex and hard working organs in the body. It performs hundreds of functions by itself. Most of these functions are important and they can disturb the functionality of the entire body, if they are not performed properly. Some of these functions include production of bile needed to digest food, monitoring and managing the blood sugar levels and removing toxins from the body. These are just some of the liver's functions. The liver has its needs too, some nutrients are important for it to function optimally. It is our job to provide these nutrients.

When the liver detoxifies the body, it doesn't just remove toxins and waste products, it also removes material that shouldn't be present in large quantities.

Toxins also don't mean only the ones that enter the body through the skin or mouth, and are called exotoxins, it also includes the toxins produced by the body. This toxins are called endotoxins. They are usually the end products of a metabolic reaction. They may then be introduced into the bloodstream by opportunistic bacteria.

Exotoxins on the other hand may enter the body through nose, skin or the mouth. Thy may be introduce through drugs, food, air pollution, household chemicals, agricultural chemicals etc.

There are two types of toxins, based on their solubility. Water soluble and fat soluble.

Fat soluble toxins are harder to remove, because they can dissolve into the body's fat content. That is why the first stage of detoxification involves making fat soluble toxins, less fat soluble.

There are 5 different chemical reactions in this first stage. The following nutrients are needed in trace quantities for the reactions:

1. Branched-chain amino acids

2. Phospholipids

3. Flavonoids

4. Vitamins B2, B3, B6, B12

5. Folate glutathione, one of the body's main antioxidants

These nutrient are needed in minute quantities but deficiency reduces the kidneys ability to remove toxins from the body.

The deficiency may be because you didn't include food that contain these nutrients in your food or because you body didn't digest the food well enough to generate the nutrients.

The first stage of detoxification makes the toxins more reactive and volatile. They are then called reactive oxygen species because increase their ability to react with other substances, including the cells of the body. It is why we need antioxidants such as coenzyme Q10, selenium, copper, zinc, manganese, thiols, pycnogemol and vitamin A, C and E. The antioxidants contracts the actions of the reactive oxygen species and prevent damages to the cells and DNA.

The reactive oxygen species are then subjected to stage 2 of the detoxification process where they become water soluble. There are 6 reactions in stage 2. After they have become water soluble, toxins can then be released into sweat, urine and stool.

Some of the nutrients required in the second stage of detoxification, especially in the amino acid conjugation reaction includes:

1. Glycine

2. Taurine

3. Cysteine

4. Ornithine

5. Methionine

6. Some Amino acids-N-acetylcysteine

7. Arginine

The liver needs the required nutrients for every reaction before it can be initiated. It also needs enbody to perform its functions, just like every other organ or part of the body. So, make sure your daily diet contains enough calories. We all get our calories from high energy carbohydrates and fats.

It the liver is unable to perform its functions, especially one like detoxification, a lot of toxins are retained in the bloodstream and other parts of the body. They can enter any part of the body and cause some damage. It is going to result in inflammatory as the body tries to fight the toxins.

If the liver becomes dysfunctional for a while, it can result in fatty liver, enlarged liver or cirrhosis of the liver.

One of the best attributed of the liver, is its ability to regenerate. It has the fastest recovery or regeneration of any organ in the body. This means that it can recover easily and fast when supplied with the right nutrients.

Overeating and poor satiety reflex

It is the job of the vagus nerve to transmit sateity signals from the stomach to the mouth. If this function is not performed properly, the individual won't be able to easily denote that he or she is full, therefore he or she will keep eating. The perso may ultimately start battling with weight problems.

A dysfunctional vagus nerve results in poor satiety diet. Obesity is one America's biggest problems. We have been dealing with this issue since the last century but we haven't found a way to combat the problem. And unknown to most people poor satiety reflex cause obesity.

Obesity in itself is an harbinger of more complicated and serious health problems such as diabetes, cancer, and heart disease to name a few.

As obesity is an harbinger of the aforementioned disease, so is poor satiety diet an harbinger of obesity.

When the vagus nerve is slow in signaling the brain that the stomach is full, it shows a dysfunction of the vagus nerve.

Note that several other factors may be responsible for obesity but mist obesity usually cones down to poor satiety reflex.

We discussed the stomachs sensitivity earlier. The ability of the stomach to expand on order to hold food. The vagus nerve is suppose to transmit to the brain when the stomach has reached its capacity. When it can't expand anymore.

It takes a while before the signal reaches the brain but it takes longer for people with poor satiety reflex. These people don't feel full after a meal after a good meal. They know the food is enough to satisfy them but they still don't feel full. This is a dysfunction in the vagus nerve.

People like these tend to keep eating until overeating become second nature. Eating an digestion is done in the rest or digest mode. In the parasympathetic side of the scope, it means that there is no work to exercise the vagus nerve

Dysfunctional microbiome

The human body has trillions of bacterial living inside it. There are much more around us and a few more on the skin. The bacteria microbiome may also act as a stressor.

The bacterial population of the body works on a balance that maintains the equilibrium. Two of the factors that influence this balance is age and dietary choices. The gut has the body's largest population of bacteria, it also makes it the likely ground zero for illness and the body's most susceptible organ.

The vagus nerve innervates the entire digestive tract. It transmits signals between the various organs wthin the digestive tract and the brain. It sends the signals that instruct the muscle walls of the intestine to push food down the channel in a process called peristalsis. The vagus nerve also transmits information from the bacterial of the gut to the cells of the small intestine.

The vagus nerve also transmits antiinflammatory signals to the gut.

Dysfunctional digestive process

The vagus nerve is involved from the beginning to the end of the digestion process. It transmits signals from the bacterial of the gut and the cells of the body to the brain, sending information about hunger and craving.

The gut bacterial fill the cravings signal that is transmitted by the vagus nerve with information about nutrients requirements.

The body needs carbohydrate and fat to generate energy, it need protein for the production of amino acids and internal protein. The body also requires other nutrients like vitamins and minerals in smaller quantities.

We ingest most of these nutrients in too while some micronutrients may be ingested as supplements.

The food enters through the mouth and takes a long journey through the entire distance of the digestive tract. The food is digested along the way while the waste products exits at the other end. It takes about 16 to 20 hours for food to digest properly. The time may vary depending on the size, age and gender of the individual. The 16 to 20 hours timeline is believed to be the best.

Anytime below 10 hours is theorized to be too short while anytime more than 24 hour so theorized as too long.

A dysfunction of the vagus nerve can hinder digestion and lead to digestive problems like constipation and diarrhea. These two are mild but common digestion problems.

The biggest problem with digestion being too quick is that the body doesn't have enough time to extract the nutrients in the food. This means that you are wasting the food.

On the other hand, if digestion is too slow, toxins can begin to build-up and bacteria may try to take advantage. It also cause leaky gut.

The digestion of food is an intricate process. After the cells of the body and gut bacteria has transmitted a signal through the vagus nerve to the brain. The brain registers the signal as hunger and we try to find something to eat. As the food sits before us or even through its aroma before it reaches our table the food startdls to estimate the salivary glands. It means the body is anticipating the meal. It is waiting and preparing for it. When you ingest the food into your mouth, before swallowing, use your teeth. Chew the food to aid your digestion. The mouth is the grinder of the digestive tract that is why our body evolved to have teeth. Chewing breaks down the food which makes it easier to move and digest them.

Chewing the food also exposes it to the taste buds. The taste buds identify and record the difference nutrients present in the food. They find out if the food contains carbohydrate, protein, and fat. The taste buds use the vagus nerve to transmit this information to the brain.

All the other organs along the digestive tract are signaled by the vagus nerve. This prepares them in anticipation of food. The pancreas, for example generates the required amount of bile and bile salt.

Another impact of chewing is an increase sensation and better enjoyment of the meal. The food tastes better. The taste buds are able to send a more detailed information to the brain. People who chwe their food also tend to eat less food than people who swallow food. The chewers are more easily satisted. It also helps that the food will digest better.

Rushing your food and not chewing it are pretty much the same thing. People who do this tend to eat more calories, make poorer dietary choices and they also have low satiety reflex.

The vagus nerves also signals the larynx and pharynx to open the through and let the model of food through. It also triggers the walls of the oesophagus to push the food down.

The food then proceeds to the stomach where the stomach acid breaks it down into indigestible fiber and marconutrient. The stomach keeps churning the food before pushing it into the small intestine. The food I'd joined in the small intestine by bile and other enzymes from the liver and gallbladder. This enzymes breakdown the food into simpler compounds. Some of the primary nutrients such as lipids, amino acid and glucose will then be absorbed into the bloodstream.

The macronutrients are then transfered into the liver where they filtered and stored to be supplied to the organs and other parts of the body.

The indigestible fiber cannot be broken down by the enzymes. It is instead moved through the small intestine, to the proximal colon of the large intestine.

The bacterial population of the large intestine then breakdown the fiber to produce minerals, vitamins and precursors for neurotransmitters and hormones. The most active element in digestion is the vagus nerve. It is always working, signaling organ after organ. For optimal functionality the vagus nerve mustn't be dealing with stress during digestion.

Digestion is a linear process. Each organ is signaled by the vagus nerve, it waits for its turn and perform its duty before the food is moved to the next organ. Being active while eating, eating on the go or multitasking while eating adds some stress to the digestive process.

We need to eat in a conducive environment with focus on the food. The vagus nerve won't be able to send the correct signals to the brain if our attention is not on the food. The added street messes with the functionality of the vagus nerve.

SECTION THREE

HOW TO MEASURE THE FUNCTIONALITY OF THE VAGUS NERVE

We can intuit that various health problems may be caused by some dysfunction of the vagus nerve. It may be true or partly true as the vagus nerve may not be solely responsible for a condition. A health condition may not even be related to the vagus nerve but all of this is just guess work and science has no room for guess work. Everything has to be proven before I can attain a degree of credibility. So even if a client exhibits some of the effects of a dysfunctional vagus nerve, the situation cannot be diagnosed as a problem with the vagus nerve until we are able to prove it. The only way to prove it is to measure the functionality of the vagus nerve.

In this chapter, we are going to discuss some techniques that can be used to measure the functionality of the vagus nerve. There are four techniques discussed in this chapter, it doesn't mean that they are the only ways to measure the functionality of the vagus nerve.

These techniques are based on measuring properties that are closely related to the activities of the vagus nerve. The four properties we are going to measure include breath pattern, heart rate, heart rate variability, bowel transit time. If these properties show a dysfunction in the vagus nerve, there is no need to panic although actions must be taken to improve the measured properties.

Breath pattern test

This test can be used as a meditation technique that allows you to breathe through the diaphragm. The test is very simple to perform.

Lie with you pack stretch straight on the floor or sit on a chair with a straight back. Place your left hand in the middle of your belly and your right hand in the middle of your chest. Then start by breathing in deeply, once. The motion will lift both the hands on your chest and stomach at equal distance, because inhalation is supposed to move the belly more than the chest. If the hand on your chest is moving faster than the hand on your belly, it means that your chest is moving more than your chest. This means that you are not breathing properly.

Several people will fall into this situation, where the chest moves more than the belly. It means they are not breathing from the diaphragm, a situation that can be corrected. It takes baby steps and daily commitments but it is doable.

Heart rate

You can use the resting heart rate to measure how healthy someone is. The average heart rate without autonomic simulation is about 100bpm, but the heat rate fluctuates between 60 to 100bpm in rest mode. It is the job of the parasympathetic nerves to keep the heart rate low. An optimal heart rate should be between 50 to 70bpms. Physical activities and exercises contribute to the heart rate. That is why athletes usually find their heart rate between 50 to 60bpm. The average healthy person's heart rate is between 60 to 70bpms. A person develops a higher risk of heart attack if the heart rate rises above 76bpms. It also increases the risk of death from any disease because the heart is weaker.

This method is based on the Heart Rate Recovery (HRR). Exercise and stress increase the heart rate but the heart rate will return to resting heart rate after the activity. How fast or slow you heart rate returns to the resting heart rate indicate the condition of the heart. The faster it takes you to recover, the healthier your heart is and vice versa. It is the responsibility of the vagus nerve to regulate the heart rate and signal for it to return to the resting heart rate. Slow recovery indicates a dysfunctional vagus nerve. High intensity exercise usually increases heart rate the most but they also tend to gradually lower the resting heart rate. You can train your heart to improve the recovery time. The standard optimal recovery should have the heart rate reduce by at least 12bpm.

You have to know your resting heart rate before you can measure your measure you recovery time. You can begin by measuring your resting heart rate a few times. There are various devices that you can use including convenient wearable technologies such as wristwatches. After discovering your heart rate, you can then start exercising and also measure your heart rate during and after workout sessions. Test you heart rate at intervals of 2 min, 4 min and 6 min after the workout. You heat rate should drop by about 24bpm at each interval. Although this depends on how rigorous the workout is your heart rate should have recovered to its resting value by the 6 min interval.

If you work out regularly and measure your heart rate recovery time after each workout, you will begin to notice and improvement in your heart arte recovery time. It means that exercise doesn't just improve your physical fitness, it also improves your cardiovascular condition. In a nutshell, exercising regularly also improves your heart condition and the response of the vagus nerve.

Heart rate variability

Out of all the methods that can be used to measure the functionality of the vagus nerve, this is the most respected and credible. It requires sophisticated equipment and a laboratory setting but you can improvise and measure it by yourself with a degree of accuracy.

The heart has four chambers; blood enters through the right and left atria and exits through the right and left ventricles.

The heartbeat occurs in two phases. The first phase involves the pumping of blood into the ventricles by the right and left atria. The second phase involves pumping blood into the pulmonary artery and the aorta, and sending deoxygenated blood to the lungs and oxygenated blood to the body cells. There is an interval after each heartbeat called the "interbeat interval." There is no electrical activity in the heart during this interval.

This moment of interval can be measured, in milliseconds to determine heart rate variability. The variation of this interval can be used to determine autonomic and cardiovascular health. a dysfunctional vagus nerve will result in less variation of the interval time.

The heart will pump at around 100bpms if no external force interferes with it, but sympathetic and parasympathetic nerves interfere with heartbeat. Sympathetic nerves influence the heart to pump at around 120bpm. This is alarmingly high because the heart is beating at a rate of two heartbeats per second. It also means the interval between heartbeats is 400 to 450 milliseconds. The interbeat interval is fairly constant with variable under 38 milliseconds, meaning that the heart rate variability is low.

Parasympathetic nerves also affect heart rate. It lowers the heart rate and therefore increases heart rate variability. Optimal heart rate is around 50 to 70bpm and the heart rate variability is usually higher.

The best time to measure your heart rate variability is when you are in rest mode. There are many tools and wearable technology that allows you to track your heart beat, one of the most popular is Fitbit Versa. We intend to measure heart rate variability and I am going to briefly talk about two tools that you can use to measure your HRR.

Inner balance by HeartMath

This tool teaches you how to measure and improve your heart rhythm. It is simple to use and can be connected to your mobile devices (both iOS and android). The aim of the tool is to help you increase your heart rate variability and attain coherence. This is HeartMath's name for optimal functioning state. You can use the connection to your device to transmit information about your conditions to your phone. It helps you to manage stressful situations.

Oura ring

Oura ring uses the photoplethysmography technique to track your interbeat intervals. It is a wearable device which allows you to access the data in real time. It monitors your conditions during training and in rest mode. It also monitors your recovery time. The best thing about oura ring is that it has an airplane mode. You can turn on the airplane mode so as not to interfere with electromagnetic frequencies (EMF).

Sesame seed bowel transit test

You can use sesame seeds to test your bowel transit time which tracks the functionality of your gut. This test is simple. You need a watch, pen and paper, water and a tablespoon of yellow or golden sesame seeds.

It works on the principle of the body's inability to digest sesame seeds and the vagus nerve's role in peristalsis. If there is a variation in the time it takes for the sesame seeds to pass through the digestive system, then the vagus nerve is dysfunctional.

To take the test, pour some sesame seeds in your cup of water, stir it and then drink the content without chewing. Note the time of ingestion on your paper. Then when you hear the call of nature, as they say. I mean when you have to go to the toilet, check your stool for sesame seeds. Mark down the time and wait until you have to go again, and then repeat the process until there is no more sesame seeds in your stool. Most of these seeds should be out by at most 20 hours, optimum time should be about 12 hours.

Any faster time than that indicates that your gut is pushing food too quickly and the vagus nerve is not functioning properly. If the experiment takes longer than 20 hours they your gut is pushing the food too slowly which is also a dysfunction of the vagus nerve.

TECHNIQUES TO ACTIVATE THE VAGUS NERVE

The body is not healthy if the vagus nerve is not functioning properly. We have discussed tests you can use to test the functionality of your vagus nerve, in the last chapter. In this chapter we are going to look at exercises to activate the vagus nerve and ensure a well-functioning autonomic nervous system.

It will probably be more efficient if you document your process, journal about your workout sessions and write about the issues and symptoms disturbing you. Acknowledge these problems and write down your goal for motivation. For example, if you are having migraine write it down and document whenever it starts, then write that you aim is to be free of migraines.

This documentation will act as motivation and also as data into the efficiency of your recovery process.

These exercises are designed to stimulate the vagus nerve through different organs and parts of the body. I have mentioned some of them earlier but here they all. They are the four components of the vagus nerve and stimulating each one has a positive effect on the other three. Here are the four components of the vagus nerve:

- Motor innervation of the larynx and pharynx

- Afferent vagus nerve signals through the visceral fibers

- Parasympathetic innervation of various organs such as the lungs, pancreas and heart

- Sensation on the skin of the central section of the ear.

Personal techniques

The following techniques and exercise can be used to manipulate the vagus nerve. They can also be performed on your own. You don't really need help from anyone, being it amateur or professional help.

Breathing Exercises

As we found out in the breathing test of the last chapter, most people are not breathing correctly. You should undertake the breathing test before trying this exercise. This first exercise is simple and effective. It is intended to teach you how to breathe properly, which activates the sympathetic nerves.

Stress alters your breathing pattern which affects the autonomic nervous system. Unlike regular people who rely on their voice to influence and wow people learn breathing techniques because it improves their ability to use their voice. Orators and singers are some of these people, consider great singers such as Celine Dion and Michael Jackson who can perform tasking songs or even dance for long period of time without seemingly losing their breath. Even more interesting are opera singers and the range they have to attain and sustain over a period of time. Most great artists including singers and instrumentalist have learnt to breathe properly, from the diaphragm. This elite club is not home to musicians alone, numerous professional athletes from basketball legend Michael Jordan, to football superstar Tom Brady or global soccer star Cristiano Ronaldo, and many other athletes all these people have something in common. They have learnt to breathe properly. It is why they are able to perform successfully in high-stress environments.

Their secret weapon is slow, calm and comforting breathing techniques. You can also learn these techniques. This theory is back up by numerous researches. Your heart rate variability can be improved using slow breathing exercises. The optimum slow breath rate may be different for each person although a research showed that reducing your breath rate to around six full breaths in a minute can improve your heart rate variability. You can still determine your own optimum slow breath rate and use it to relief stress. Here is the exercise in simple steps.

- Sit up straight without resting your back on anything

- Exhale fully to push out all the air in your lungs.

- Place your left hand on the center of your belly and your right hand on the center of your chest.

- Breathe in deeply through your nose for about 5 to 7 seconds and feel your belly moving.

- Hold the breath for about 2 to 3 seconds.

- Then exhale through your mouth and feel your belly fall.

- Hold that breathe without letting any air into your lungs for 2 to 3 seconds.

- Repeat the 4th and 7th step during each set for as many times as comfortable.

Practice this exercise for about 5 minutes every day. You can also practice it multiple times per day, if you have the time. Make sure you perform it in private so that you won't be disturbed. You can also work on your focus so that you can try it pretty much anywhere without your attention wavering.

This exercise improves your stress levels, mood and general wellbeing. Even if you don't have a lot of time on your hands, a little effort will have considerable effect.

Sleeping breath patterns and mouth tapping

The earlier exercise is about when we are awake and can make conscious efforts to control our breath. Sleeping is different, we have no conscious control. Experts instruct that the body needs about 7 to 8 hours of sleep every night and during this period we take about 7,200 breaths. That is 1/3 of our daily breath, taken while we are asleep. So, why not try to influence our sleeping breath pattern and improve its efficiency. In order words, we can learn to breathe optimally during sleep. The breath pattern is also a habit and we are likely to fall into the most familiar and in this case poor breathing patterns while asleep. Take something like obstructive sleep apnea which is a creation of habit and a growing social problem. It has negative effect on the health. The patient will not know if he has sleep apnea unless someone sleeping tells him or he records himself sleeping. It includes snoring and maybe not breathing for a few moments during sleep. This is due to a dysfunctional vagus nerve. It is also stressful to the body which is choking each time you stop breathing. Of course you can attribute the issue to excess weight and they may reduce if you lose weight but there is the likelihood of it rearing its head once in a while.

If you stop breathing through your nose the mouth immediately takes charge. This allows you to maintain your breath but it has long term side effects. The lack of airflow in the lungs affects the ceiling walls of the nasal passage and the microbes of the nose. It results in post-nasal drip, long-term obstruction of the nasal passages and increased allergies.

One technique that you can use to combat this is mouth tapping. It is very simple and all you need is a piece of paper. When you want to sleep, tape the paper to your mouth, using it to seal it shut.

It is more difficult to use the diaphragm when breathing through the mouth than it is when breathing though the nose. That is why breathing through the nose is second nature. It improves the functionality of the vagus nerve. You can combine mouth tap and breathing exercises to maximum effect.

Reduce your exposure to evening blue light

The body has the ability to adapt to the changes in wavelength of lighting at different points in of a day. From the warm sunlight of the morning coming from the rising sun and usually with red/yellow wavelengths, to the sharper blue light of noon and the red/yellow hue of the evening due to the setting sun. The body reacts to these, secrete hormones and transmit signals that inform us what time of the day it is. Exposure to blue light in the evening signals the body that the time is noon. It reduces the production of the hormone called melatonin. Melatonin is secreted by the body at evening time to help us relax. There are several modern devices with screens that emit light with blue wavelength such as a mobile phone, television and laptop etc.

Modern technology will also save us, as some devices now have blue-light filters built into them. There are also many apps that you can download to filter blue light on your mobile devices (both iOS and android).

A simple solution is to reduce your screen-time at night. Read a book instead or hang out with friends instead of staring at your phone.

Turn off your electronics devices at night or during rest time

You shouldn't have to worry about the outside world and any form of distraction while resting. Sleeping at night or resting during the day relieves stress and refreshes the body. Electronic devices such as phones, PCs and television are one of the biggest distractions we have today. Turn them off while you are sleeping so that you can shut out the outside world and rest comfortably. Our phones are usually the main culprit. Turn it off or turn on the airplane mood whenever you need to rest. You can also try charging it in a separate room or putting it on silent so that incoming calls won't disturb you.

Eat dinner early

A lot of people eat their dinner late and take to bed soon after. This can impair the proper digestion of food. It can also break up your sleep and reduce sleep quality. You should have at least 2 hours between your dinners and sleep time. When you eat or drink late, you are going to end up waking in the middle of the night to visit the toilet. This may happen numerous times every night and it disrupts your sleep.

Care for your sleeping space

The quality of your sleep is affected by the hygiene of your bedroom or sleeping space. Since the quality of your sleep affects your ability to perform daily functions and overall wellbeing, then you must consider every factor that may affect your sleep.

If your bedroom is dirty or disorganized, it will always creep into your thoughts and discourage your spirit anytime you see it. You are going to see it every night and every morning since you will be sleeping and waking up in it. It is going to create a negative energy that affects you the most at strategic moments, when you wake up in the morning and when you are going to sleep at night. It will disturb our sleep at night and your mood and focus in the morning. This is because of the additional stress it causes that counteracts the effects of the parasympathetic nerves.

Try to ensure a clean, tidy and organized bedroom. Remember that it doesn't just affect your sleep, it also affects your mood as you wake up in the morning and prepare take on the day.

Sleep on your side

The Circulation Journal published a survey in 2008. The aim of the research was to determine the effect of sleeping positions on people who have coronary heart diseases. According to the research, sleeping on your side is better for the test group and

A 2008 study by Yang et al. published in *Circulation Journal* compared the HRV levels of different sleep positions. The study was done to determine the best position for patients dealing with coronary artery disease compared to those without any blockages in their coronary arteries. The researchers found lying on your back is the worst position for HRV levels, both for test and control patients, while lying on either side showed significant improvement in HRV levels. Most interestingly, sleeping on the right side was found to be the best for vagal modulation, especially in the control group and anyone in general while sleeping on your back is generally bad for anybody.

It is not just about sleeping on your back; the basis of the research can also apply to lying on your back. The major difference between lying on your back and sleeping on your back is consciousness and time. Sleeps usually take hours and lying down may take a shorter periods of time. This means that lying down on your back for extended period of time will have the same effect as sleeping on your back.

Both sleeping on your back and laying on your back affects the vagus nerve while sleeping or lying on your side positively impacts the vagus nerve. This is due to the airway, which is important to proper breathing. When you are on your back, gravity pushes the tongue back and it ends up blocking the airway. The likelihood of these happening when you are on your side is very unlikely. It doesn't matter if you are lying on your right side or left side.

Since most people sleep on their back and it is most likely second nature to them, a creation of habit, you need to teach yourself to sleep on your back. One simple and effective option is to place a pillow in-between your thighs as you fall asleep. It makes it harder for you to roll back onto your back. The pillow will most likely fall off but you will keep repeating it until your body becomes used to having a pillow there and maintaining the position. You can remove thi pillow over time.

Chanting and humming

Remember that vagus nerve innervates the laryngeal muscles and other voluntary muscles. You can manipulate these muscles and use them to influence the vagus nerve. These muscles signal the brain through the vagus nerve and this network can be manipulated. Take one of these voluntary muscles for example; the laryngeal muscles can be activated by chanting and humming. This activity raises the pitch of the voice, strengthens the vocal chords and reduces tension. The signal is sent to the brainstem through the recurrent and superior laryngeal branches of the vagus nerve. This ensures that the vagus nerve itself is stimulated through vibration, since it is the road network or to put it in another way, it contains the connection that transmits the signal.

There are various words or syllable you cans use such as Ameen, Amen, Om and Amin. All this words are related to religion. I suggest using the Hindu syllable "om". When you recite "om" aloud, it produces a deep vibration in your throat. In Hinduism "Om" is a spiritual syllable with a similar spiritual role as the other syllables that I mentioned.

These words generate a vibration deep in the throat that activates the vocal chords and laryngeal muscles. It other words, it stimulates a part of the vagus nerve but if you try it over a long period of time with strength and volume, the impact is more powerful and it extends to other parts of the vagus nerve.

Chanting allows us to relax and stop worrying. When the body enters relaxation mode, it can improve the activities of the autoimmune system, the management of inflammation and digestion.

You can try chanting or humming several times in a day. You can set aside time to meditate and add chanting and humming exercises or you can just use it during times of excessive stress.

Chanting and humming decreases the activation of the sympathetic muscles, meaning that it reduces stress and the activator of stressor hormones.

Start practicing chanting and humming, retain the habit and you will reap the benefits soon enough.

Using the gag reflex

Another muscle innervated by the vagus nerve is the pharyngeal muscles. The pharyngeal muscles can also be stimulated in a process similar to the one used to stimulate the laryngeal. The gag reflex is designed to prevent us from choking. Any object that unknowingly (to us) enters the mouth activates a signal when it touches the soft surfaces of the back roof of the mouth (called the soft palate). The signal is transmitted through the vagus nerve to the brainstem and then to three different cranial nerve's motor aspects. The first cranial nerve that receives the signal is the pharyngeal muscles located at the back of the throat. The job of the pharyngeal muscles is to prevent the object from passing through into the deeper parts of the body. If the object makes it pass the pharyngeal muscles it may not even make it pass the airway, where it can choke the person to death. The pharyngeal muscles don't work alone. After the pharyngeal muscles block the airway and prevent the object from passing through, the two other cranial nerves that received the signal, the cranial nerve 5 and the cranial nerve 12 keep the jaw open as the tongue tries to push out the subject.

This process is unconscious and controlled by the central nervous system but we can voluntarily activate the vagus nerve in other to activate and manipulate the vagus nerve.

The easiest and most convenient time to do this is when brushing your teeth. Since you are already thrusting an object (your toothbrush) into your mouth, and according to dental experts, it is also healthy to brush to times per day, in the morning and before going to bed at night. So let's say that you can try to manipulate the vagus nerve by activating the gag reflex twice a day, in the morning and at night.

All you need to do is stick the toothbrush deep into your mouth until it slightly touches the roof of the back of your throat. This is where the soft palate is located and touching it will stimulate it which in turn stimulates the vagus nerve.

Instead of just centralizing the action, you can stimulate the soft palate closer to the sides of your mouth.

Gargling

Gargling simply involves pouring a mixture in your mouth (usually water, water and salt or mouth wash) and swirling it around vigorously. It is healthy, kills the germs in the mouth (the mouth is one of our body parts with the most germs), it also helps to combat mouth odor. To our advantage it can also be used to stimulate the vagus nerve. Similar to the gag reflex, it triggers the three pharyngeal muscles located at the back of our throat.

It also shares another similarity with activating the gag reflex, the best time to practice gargling is after brushing your teeth, both in the morning and at night.

Mild gargling won't cut it, you need to gargle with vigor until tears begin to sting your eyes. At this point, signals have been transmitted to the brain through the vagus nerve. The brainstem also sends signals that activate adjacent nuclei such as the superior salivary nucleus. This activates the glands at the eye which produce tears. I hope you get that tearing up is the aim of this exercise. You can only know that the exercise worked and the vagus nerve has been well stimulated when tears begin to form.

In order to increase the efficiency of the exercise, don't use ordinary water. Add a little oil to the water or salt especially Himalayan pink salt. It cleans up the mouth and throat.

Cryotherapy or cold exposure

Cold exposure or cryotherapy as it is called scientifically is an emerging science for activating the parasympathetic cells.

It is similar to jumping into a lake or any other body of cold water. The cold hits suddenly and penetrates into the core as the body starts to shiver and the teeth starts to clatter. If you have ever tried this, you will know that the breaths also become very shallow and quick, because the sympathetic nerves have been activated and you are in fight or flight mode.

While this is action activates the sympathetic nerves, as we have seen, it is also be used to activate the parasympathetic nerves. The situation activates the sympathetic nerves on the short-term but the parasympathetic nerves take control over the long-term.

This principle is applied in cryotherapy, which exposes you to continuous acute cold and you start to learn how to regulate your breath as the process continues. This is good for the vagus nerve and it also combats inflammation.

For another dramatic and common occurrence that demonstrates the healing power of cold exposure, consider why we hold cold substances to bruises. This is very common with athletes but you can also see it with anyone who bruises a body part. The cold activates the vagus nerve and you can incorporate the principle into your daily routine. Some people take a cold bath (or should I call it soak) in a tub filled with water and ice. They dip themselves into this cold water filled tub and stay in it for a while. If these seem extreme for you, you can try incorporating cold shower into your morning bath. I am not talking about an extreme cold water bath, I mean letting cold water run through your head, the back of your neck and the rest of your entire body after your initial bath and before leaving the bathroom.

It will shock your body and reduce your breathing to shallow deep breaths. You will experience the symptoms that we discussed earlier but mildly. You must aim to regulate your breathing, by trying to reduce the peed of your breath while reducing its depth. Training your body to breath in the cold strengthens your vagus nerve and parasympathetic nerves.

Start by having a minute of cold shower and try regulating your breathing pattern. As you get better in the one minute period, you can gradually increase the time period by a minute or two until you are satisfied.

Exercising and working out

The human body was designed for movement. The legs are built to run, while the hands and the shape and positioning of the remaining parts of our body is designed to maintain balance. Even a machine will rust and break then if it is not used regularly, not to talk of the human body. Our body needs daily exercise at the least and physical fitness workout, if you can. It is more than a physical fitness thing. Working out is an effective way to burn fat and calories. It also helps to maintain the blood sugar level.

Many of us live a sedentary life style. You wake up in the morning and leave your house in a car. You get to work and your job involves sitting down. Then after office hours, you get back in the car which takes you home, where you resume sitting until you are ready to go to bed and repeat the circle on the next day. There is some variety but this give a general idea of most peoples live. The body is meant to be moved and exercised. Running is one of the easiest and most basic form of exercise. Science has proven that running has a massive benefit for the human body.

Running and other exercises also benefits the vagus nerve. This exercised induce stress on the body and increase the heart rate. This stimulates both the sympathetic and parasympathetic nerves. It also strengthens the heart, teaching it to pump more blood.

While the stress stimulates the sympathetic nerves, recovery stimulated the parasympathetic nerves. Recovery also teaches how to regulate breath patterns

We should exercise regularly, daily to be exact. The stress induced and recovery trains the body and vital organs every time. The vagus nerve is not exempted. It also teaches how to handle stress and improves the recovery time for any stressful event.

Yoga or Pilates

Yoga and Pilates are two of those exercises that act as both work out and meditation. It strengthens both the body and mind. It also helps you regulate your breath. Both exercises require you to eliminate external stress and influence. They both involve voluntary breathing techniques.

Yoga sessions are designed to teach you how to how to control your breathing, that is why they begin and end with slow deep belly breathing exercises. The exercise themselves engage the body in various physical stresses. It is designed to stress the muscles and this impact can be improved by adding heat and humidity. That is why practices like hot yoga and the various new twists to yoga and Pilates are turning up every day.

The body can improve and function better if you learn to maintain these breathing practices used during yoga and Pilates, when under stress. Breathing is one of the main outer manifestations of stress, when you train yourself to control your breathing, then you can start to control your body's reaction to a stressful environment. You will be able to maintain your composure and better handle stress.

Both breathing exercises stimulate the vagus nerve. The breathing exercise are even more effective because they paired with exercise that target various stressors of the body.

Pilates itself was founded with the goal of helping people combat stress by learning to breath properly. Stress changes our breathing; it reduces our ability to breathe properly. When you practice pilates, you begin to take control of your breathing under stress.

Your diet

Food is not just a way to satiate hunger. The nutrients present in food is digested and used to supply energy, develop and maintain the body. We have started to improve our understanding of food and its impact on the human body. There are foods that are essential to the body because of the nutrients they contain. There are also foods that are important by needed only in small quantity because the nutrients they contain are needed in small quantity. There are also foods that we need to avoid, especially if the person has a condition, these are also because of the nutrients present in such food item. This is a simple generalization of nutrition but understanding this gets you in the door.

On the cases of food that we have to avoid, the nutrients present in such foods affect the digestion and the cells and organs of the body. It may also increase inflammation. While fat and carbs get a bad rep, processed food, generally is the enemy.

These foods contain additives and other chemicals that are harmful to the body. These chemicals may residual herbicides and pesticides, hormones, preservatives and so on.

While everyone should avoid these food items, people with health conditions should go out of their way in order to stay away from these food items. It can elevate their condition.

You still have to eat so it is not complete to only tell you what food items you shouldn't eat. I must also tell you about the ones you can eat. The idea is to go natural and healthy. Organic and locally grown food because they are likely to contain less chemicals. You should also switch to grass feed meat and organic nuts.

These are just few options and as much as I would love to discuss the food choices, I am afraid I can't dwell too long on this. You can find information online on healthy food choices. I love visiting www.healthline.com so maybe you should try it. They have many great advices on dietary choices. Oh that word "diet", we were walking up to it and now we have arrived there. There are several diets available today, examples include keto diet, paleo diet, vegan diet, autoimmune paleo diet and much more. Whichever diet plan you undertake should depend on your goal and health condition. Instead of trying generalized diet plans, you can also work with professionals to create your individualized diet plan. Your personal diet plan should cater to your need, income, preferences and health status.

I will tell you one thing though, reduce your visit to the grocery store and use a farmers market instead. The products of a farmers market are fresher and healthier. You will also find variety of options and fruits and vegetables that may not be available at the grocery store.

After our brief discussion on dietary choices, which is incomplete like I said. Try to read a book on nutrition, in order to better understand how your diet affects your health.

Let's talk about of focus in this book and this chapter in particular, diet and the vagus nerve. How we can use diet to stimulate the vagus nerve and increase bits functionality. Acetylcholine (ACh), the neurotransmitter has been mentioned numerous times in this book. It is very important to the vagus nerve. ACh is the main neurotransmitter used by the vagus nerve to transmit signals. This means that the vagus nerve can't function properly without it. ACh is produced in the body but the nutrients required to produce it must be provided through food. I hope you are getting were I am headed. You need to eat foods that contain the nutrients required to produce ACh. ACh is produced from acetyl coenzyme A and choline.

Acetyl coenzyme A is produced from free fatty acid and glucose. This means that you must include foods that contain these ingredients in your diet (even if it is in small fraction because only a little bit is needed). Free fatty acid is generated from the digestion of fat, while glucose is generated from the digestion of carbohydrate. These gives you a lot of option, you just have to add some fat and carbohydrate to your diet.

The second nutrient required is choline. Choline cannot be produced by the body so you have to directly ingest food items that contain choline. Examples of such food items are proteins such as soy, beef, turkey liver, chicken and egg yolks have the highest supply of choline.

You can also improve the functionality of the vagus nerve by resting it. The vagus nerve is involved from the ingestion of food to the release of waste products from the body. You can give it some time off by reducing the workload. You can rest the vagus nerve by fasting. Intermittent fasting is common and effective. One of the indicators of an improving vagus nerve is an improved heart rate variability and intermittent fasting has been proven to improve heart rate variability.

Intermittent fasting is based on having about 6 to 8 hours between meals. It also involves counting and monitoring your calorie intake.

Taking supplements

There are some nutrients that are needed by the body in minute quantities but are not available in the food items that make up the bulk of our diet. For majority of us of diet is made up of a particular class of food and essential but trace nutrients such as vitamins and minerals are not being adequately supplied to the body. These nutrients may be needed by organs or cells or even the microbiome of the digestive tract. Supplementation is a great way to provide the body with such nutrients. Supplements are not to be taken just because, that is why some people believe that they are a waste of money. Only people who are deficient in certain nutrients can take supplements in order to boast their body's supply of such nutrients. The only way to know if you are deficient is through medical tests and diagnoses provided by health professionals such as doctors, nutritionists and the like.

There are still some still some supplements that most of the general public needs, but even that opinion requires the counsel of a professional.

So no mater your condition, your aim for using a supplement or the effect that supplement is suppose of have, don't self-prescribe. Consult a professional, preferably one who knows your medical history.

Mindfulness

Mindfulness is giving extra focus and attention to your tasks and environment. It allows you to enjoy and appreciate your surroundings. You can do this in alone times or before beginning a task.

A lot of us are guilty of not being mindful. We go through life, from one activity to another without paying attention to what is happening around us. We drive on auto pilot and don't pay attention to the little things. The little things matter and they have unimaginable power to relax the mind, body and soul.

Without mindfulness, we won't be able to stay a 100 percent committed to our responsibilities because we won't see the whole picture. We tend to ignore the things that we believe are unnecessary.

Mindfulness is a full-on and gradual turnaround from before. We begin to consider every factor and their impact. We become more grateful.

The main problem is the stress and fast paced lifestyle of the modern world. Professionals are the most susceptible to this, as the sympathetic nerves are in overdrive keeping people in constant fight or flight modes.

Mindfulness makes use of breathing practices and planning to accomplish tasks and improve your focus. The parasympathetic nerves are in charge when we become mindful. It is a way of stimulating the vagus nerve. It also improves your attention to detail and ability to complete a task effectively.

Mindfulness is not just about work. You can be mindful in every aspect of your life, even in pleasure. Mindful relaxation allows the body to properly rejuvenate, revamp and refuel. Mindful eating allows you to enjoy your food, detect when you are full and prevent overeating.

Since the sympathetic nerves are in charge and the body is in rest mode. It allows the organs and every part of the body to prioritize relaxation.

Mindfulness also involves the reduction of multitasking. Multitasking may seem like a good idea to quickly complete multiple tasks at the same time but it also makes sure that you are not fully committed to any task. You risk missing vital steps that may require you to repeat the task, therefore negating the time that you saved earlier.

As said earlier, mindfulness has positive part on the body. It uplifts the body, the mind and the spirit.

Meditation

Meditation is about being attentive to your thoughts. The brain is a very dynamic organ designed to find connections between random thoughts and acts. The aim of meditation is to allow the mind wander unhindered. You stop trying to lead or control your thinking and let your brain set the course. There are different types of mediation and one could write an entire book on meditation alone.

Out of all the different types of meditation, the most efficient ones for stimulating the vagus nerve are the types that focus on breathing patterns and techniques. These types of meditation help to improve heart rate and therefore strengthen the vagus nerve.

I also want to talk about meditating the right way. This can create a paradox. According to a research published by the international journal of psychophysiology, the idea of perfect meditation may be an illusion that ultimately reduces the effects of meditation. The study found out the patients who labeled themselves as perfectionists and tried to perfect their meditation couldn't attain any improvement in the heart rate variability. Patients who aren't trying to perfect their meditation on the other hand, ended up with improved heart rate variability.

The major difference between the two groups is control issues. The perfectionist group tried to control their meditation, which is wrong. The whole idea of meditation is to let go of control. This doesn't mean that there is you don't need to practice meditation, you do. There is an art to meditating and you have to learn it.

The best option is to find a teacher or guru, but medication should be an in the moment activity. You need to have your teacher or instructor with you in the early stages of your meditation. It is not a problem if you can't make it to a meditation class. I believe that meditation should be a private act anyway. There are numerous mediation books and audios you can buy and listen to online or in your neighborhood bookshop. Find an instructor you can trust or the techniques you are comfortable with. You can try different trainers and techniques until you find the right one. Nobody will hold you. You just need to approach meditation with an open mind and spirit before you can reap the benefits. Try something a few times before you chalk it off as a failed experiment. Better still, substitute techniques, performing each one a few times a week or return to a long abandoned meditation technique later in the future. Give it one more try.

If you are wondering how you will know if a mediation technique works for you, trust me you will know. If you are still in doubt you can use a tool that measures heart rate variability, since your main aim for meditating is to improve your heart rate variability and therefore harness the healing power of the vagus nerve. I believe that at least two of such tools were mentioned in the last chapter. You can also find a different tool on the internet if the ones mentioned are not convenient for you.

Exposure to sunlight

The human body and sunlight is linked. We absorb sunlight through the skin and eyes. It is how understand the hour of the day and in the olden days, it was how they found their way to their destination. The body must be exposed to sunlight but it must be at a moderate level because excessive sunlight is damaging to the body and health. If you have ever spent a day or a couple of days indoor, you are of the feeling of the sun hitting your face, when you finally come out into the light.

Sunlight affects the functionality of the body on the cellular level. It also affects heart rate variability. During the day, lights of ultraviolet, green, violet and blue wavelengths are best for the eyes and skin, but in the morning or evening lights of yellow, red and infrared wavelengths are better. The sun automatically provides them. Indoor lights, however cannot switch wavelength like the sun does.

Getting the required wavelength at the right time improves your heart arte variability. This means you have to expose yourself at different intervals for the different wavelengths. Spending the long period of time under the sun may lead to sun burn, so you have to be more strategic. You can get outside for some minutes several times a day.

Companionship and Laughter

Many recent studies have proven that laughter is good for the body. Some of these studies insinuate that laughter may increase our lifespan. Even if you don't believe all this, you can't deny how good it feels to laugh. Laughter releases a feel good chemical into the body. Remember the last time you had fun and laugh without care. The impact was extending beyond that moment. Even after the event your mood remains elevated. Even the memory of that moment can lift your mood.

Laughter can also improve your heart rate variability. When we have a big laugh, it tends to come from the diaphragm. We already know how important the diaphragm is to breathing properly. The diaphragm is being exercised and that is good for breathing and the vagus nerve.

So next time you are at a social event enjoy your laugh. Better yet, hang out at locations that make you laugh, watch a comedy or hang around people with positive energy. You can also bring laughter into your yoga classes. Laugh with your mates as yoga can also elevate the mood and improve heart rate variability. Laughter does both of these also and you will be combining laughter and yoga for positive effect.

Yoga classes also offer companionship. You can laugh alone in your home. Enjoy a movie and listen to a stand-up comedy track but human beings are social animal and it is going to get lonely in there someday. The warmth and company of other people is essential to our health. It has consequences on the wellbeing of the body, soul and mind. From the beginning of our history, we have always been social animals. Our myths and religious doctrines may start history with one person but a companion always appears soon enough. The presence of others uplifts our mood.

In this modern world of connectivity, with the world now a global village, people couldn't be lonelier. It may be due to the reduction of physical contact and face to face interactions.

This doesn't mean you have to desperately hang around people that try to bring you down or don't share your values. There are billions of people out there. I know only a fraction of those people live near you but you will find your people.

People you can connect to and share your experience with, people whose presence improves your mood and ultimately, your health, people you can laugh, throw your head back and relax with. I am not trying to create a romantic and incorrect idea of a relationship because every relationship has its up and downs.

When you are with this kind of people even mundane things are funnier, memories are lovelier and events are more enjoyable.

The only remedy to loneliness is to reconnect with society. It is not going to be easy especially if you are the extremely introverted type. One of the funniest things about making friends is that it may actually be easier than we think. Friend ships are built on similarity of interests and values. How about you consider what you enjoy and value, and then find somewhere that people who share your interests and values would go. People who love sport would visits stadiums or watch games in bars, both are stuffier and louder than the comfort of your house but they have people who likely share your interest. That is why you are visiting. If you enjoy comedy visit a comedy clubs, watch a movie at the cinema once in a while instead of always spending your time on Netflix and if you are the type who loves working out, join a gym or sport club.

Think about all those carefree jovial and always laughing people you may hate but are actually jealous of. Consider how happy and good they feel and look. That is what laughter does to you. As I said earlier, laughter release feel good chemicals into the bloodstream. The name of this chemical is endorphin.

The healing power of music

Music is one of the strangest and most wonderful invention men as ever created. The same can be said of most art but music is very special and on a field of its own. It doesn't matter if you understand the lyrics, or even if it is just instrumentals without lyrics or chanting, music has a charming and healing effect on the human mind, body and spirit. Think about the effect a lullaby has on a baby that doesn't even understand words yet. It extends our limits and opens up new horizons. It also empowers the body exceed expectations. There is this story of this cellist, Pablo Casals. He had rheumatoid arthritis and emphysema. Some of the symptoms include inability to keep the back straight or stand straight, inability to work unaided and unsteady hands, among other things. Every morning, Mr. Casals would shuffle and drag himself to his piano. He would unclench his hands and start playing Bach's "Wohltemperierte Klavier."

During this, his breathing will become more relaxed and his back would straighten. He will give himself completely to this music, humming and playing with great skill and without care. He would then move to the more upbeat Brahms concerto and play it without skipping a beat. After his session, his body will become freer and stronger. He will be able to walk unaided and stand tall. He then enjoys his breakfast and goes for a walk. That is the power of music.

While most of use can't play the exquisite musical pieces or even own or play the piano, we have devices that play music and we can enjoy a sing along. Whether in the privacy of our bathroom or in our car, we love singing along to music. Music relaxes the body and triggers the parasympathetic nerves of the vagus nerve.

There have been several studies on the effect of music on patients. One study by Chung et al. in 2010 monitored cancer patients exposed to a music therapy session of 2 hours. The patients experienced improvement in their heart rate variability. This means that music has an effect on the parasympathetic nerves and the vagus nerve.

For your own experiment, try listening to music when you are tired or stressed. Listen to music before starting your day, at the end of your day or anytime in between. Sing along to the music, dance to it. You don't need to know the entire lyrics, have a great voice or try intricate and complex dance moves. You just need to have some fun. Let your body relax while the music takes control. I want to leave in with the lyrics of one song. Music- it heals your body, heals your soul, heals your spirit. Get in the music.

Professional techniques that activates the vagus nerve

The following techniques stimulate the vagus nerve but you can't perform them by yourself. They require professional attention. For some of these techniques, you may invite the professional into your home or you may visit a professional health center. You might prefer these techniques because of the presence of an expert.

Chiropractic therapy

Due to a more sedentary life style, many people are dealing with back pain and a mechanical neck. The modern work place requires us to sit in front of a screen for hours. The way we spend our spare time is also similar. The muscles become stiff because they have not been fully stretched for a long period of time.

Chiropractors work on the joints, muscles and the pain. A reduction in pain is good for breathing and the vagus nerve. It also heals and renews the joint.

Massage Therapy

Many people undergo massage therapy sessions. It is great way for the body to relax and ease tensions on the skin. What the body feels after a massage can hardly be described but I will try. The body feels refreshed, renewed, uplifted, it breathes deeper etc. there are many adjectives to describe a massage and one person's will be different from another's.

A massage stimulates the parasympathetic nerves. It also improves heat rate variability. There are several massage techniques available out there; even electronic devices are getting in the game with the invention of massage chairs and other devices.

Auricular Acupuncture

In the earliest chapter, we discus some of the control points of the vagus nerve. I mentioned four control points. One of these control points is the skin of the central anterior ear, the auricle. The parts of the auricle that can be stimulated include the tragus, the crus of the helix and the concha. Acupuncture sends a signal form this control point. The signal will be transmitted through the auricular branch of the vagus nerve. Therefore it stimulates the vagus nerve.

Research shows that patients battling with chronic pain, epilepsy, depression, inflammation and anxiety benefit from acupunctural stimulation of the vagus nerve. Above all, acupuncture is a safe practice without any significant side effect.

A new type of therapy using electrical stimulation to stimulate the vagus nerve is also growing. This therapy requires an electrical device to be surgically implanted directly into the vagus nerve. This therapy does pretty much the same thing as auricular acupuncture but it is not as safe. The science is still blurry and many consequences are unknown.

Visceral Manipulation

This is very effective but it is not as common as the others. It requires indelible training and technique before it can be performed properly. It involves the gentle physical manipulation of the abdomen and the organs located there. The practitioners who usually perform it include chiropractors, osteopaths and naturopaths.

They gentle massage the abdomen to locate areas of decrease, stalled or altered motion.

The aim is to increase the flow of blood to the organs in the manipulated area. These include organs like small and large intestine, spleen, pancreas, stomach, gallbladder, kidney and the liver. All of these organs are innervated by the vagus nerve. The signal for more blood flow is transmitted through the vagus nerve. When the organs are manipulated properly and blood flow is increased, physical restriction will be altered, ensuring that the organs also benefit from the action.

CONCLUSION

This book is not the beginning or the end of the discussion on the vagus nerve. It was intended to introduce you to the vagus nerve, show how it affects you and how you can harness its healing power. It is still just a starting point, but it is easy to read and understand. Maybe after you have read this book and you have tried the exercises, it will spark more interest in you. The vagus nerve is not a new discovery, most people are just not awae about it. The few who are aware can't fathom the extent of its impact. Nobody really can and that's is not a bad thing.

Harnessing the hidden power of the vagus nerve is not a contradiction of medical science, neither is it declaring war on therapy, but like every genuine and powerful healing principle, it is to be applied along with modern medicine. To pick up the slack when medicine wavers or takes a generalized and counterproductive approach to some cases.

REFERENCES

Dr. Navaz Habib, Activate your vagus nerve: Unleash your body's natural ability to overcome- gut sensitivities, autoimmunity, inflammation, anxiety, brain fog and depression

Stanley Rosenberg, Acessing the healing power of the vagus nerve: self-help exercises for anxiety, depression, trauma and autism

Beth Spindler, Yoga therapy for fear: treating anxiety, depression and rage with the vagus nerve and other techniques

Kaminoff, L. (2009) Talk given at the breathing project, New York.